Posttraumatic Epilep

Posttraumatic Epilepsy
Basic and Clinical Aspects

Carrie R. Jonak
Division of Biomedical Sciences, School of Medicine,
University of California, Riverside, CA, United States

Allison R. Peterson
Division of Biomedical Sciences, School of Medicine,
University of California, Riverside, CA, United States

Devin K. Binder
Center for Glial-Neuronal Interactions,
Division of Biomedical Sciences, School of Medicine,
University of California, Riverside, CA, United States

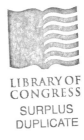

ELSEVIER

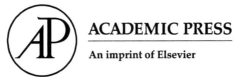
ACADEMIC PRESS
An imprint of Elsevier

Academic Press is an imprint of Elsevier
125 London Wall, London EC2Y 5AS, United Kingdom
525 B Street, Suite 1650, San Diego, CA 92101, United States
50 Hampshire Street, 5th Floor, Cambridge, MA 02139, United States
The Boulevard, Langford Lane, Kidlington, Oxford OX5 1GB, United Kingdom

Notices
Knowledge and best practice in this field are constantly changing. As new research and experience broaden our understanding, changes in research methods, professional practices, or medical treatment may become necessary.

Practitioners and researchers must always rely on their own experience and knowledge in evaluating and using any information, methods, compounds, or experiments described herein. In using such information or methods they should be mindful of their own safety and the safety of others, including parties for whom they have a professional responsibility.

To the fullest extent of the law, neither the Publisher nor the authors, contributors, or editors, assume any liability for any injury and/or damage to persons or property as a matter of products liability, negligence or otherwise, or from any use or operation of any methods, products, instructions, or ideas contained in the material herein.

ISBN 978-0-323-90099-7

For information on all Academic Press publications
visit our website at https://www.elsevier.com/books-and-journals

Publisher: Nikki P. Levy
Acquisitions Editor: Joslyn T. Chaiprasert-Paguio
Editorial Project Manager: Barbara L. Makinster
Production Project Manager: Niranjan Bhaskaran
Cover Designer: Matthew Limbert

Typeset by STRAIVE, India

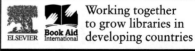

Working together
to grow libraries in
developing countries

www.elsevier.com • www.bookaid.org

Dedication

To my mother, Yolanda, the strongest person I know

To my husband, Paul, whose love, patience, and support gives me hope

Carrie R. Jonak

To my husband, Nick, whose love and endless support has strengthened me throughout my academic journey

Allison R. Peterson

To the towering legacy and inspiring examples of Wilder Penfield and A. Earl Walker—two neurosurgeon-scientists who made seminal contributions to the field of posttraumatic epilepsy among many others and who have stimulated many brain explorers that follow to fruitfully combine neuroscience and neurosurgery

Devin K. Binder

Contents

Preface   xi
Acknowledgments   xiii

1. History of posttraumatic epilepsy

Overview   1
Hippocrates   1
The Middle Ages and Renaissance   3
Trephination to craniotomy: Early surgical approaches
    to epilepsy   4
Early pioneers in cortical localization   7
Rise of neurology and neurosurgery in parallel
    in the 1870s and 1880s   12
Toward the 20th century and localization-related epilepsy   17
References   24

2. Epidemiology of posttraumatic epilepsy

Overview   29
Military injuries   29
Civilian injuries   34
Risk factors   36
Natural history   38
References   39

3. Neuropathology of posttraumatic epilepsy

Overview   43
Wilder Penfield   43
Penfield's description of oligodendroglia   49
Glial alterations in neurological disease: Early concepts   52
From neurocytology to neuropathology: Toward understanding
    of the cicatrix   53
Penfield and Foerster: Toward neuropathology
    of posttraumatic epilepsy   56
Penfield's other contributions   61
Toward more modern histopathology: TBI to PTE?   63
References   64

4. Clinical trials of agents to prevent posttraumatic epilepsy

Overview	67
Vietnam prophylaxis program	67
Carbamazepine study	68
Phenytoin studies	68
Valproate study	69
Magnesium study	70
Levetiracetam studies	70
Perspective	71
References	71

5. Surgical treatment of posttraumatic epilepsy

Overview	73
Arthur Earl Walker	73
Modern series of surgical treatments of posttraumatic epilepsy	81
Case example: Surgical treatment of posttraumatic epilepsy	84
Perspective	89
References	89

6. Animal models of traumatic brain injury

Overview	91
Fluid percussion injury	91
Controlled cortical impact injury	91
Weight drop injury	92
Penetrating ballistic-like brain injury	94
Blast-induced traumatic brain injury	96
Undercut traumatic brain injury	97
References	98

7. Incidence of posttraumatic epilepsy in animal models of traumatic brain injury

Overview	105
Fluid percussion injury	105
Controlled cortical impact injury	108
Weight drop injury	108
Penetrating ballistic-like brain injury	108
Blast-induced traumatic brain injury	110
Undercut traumatic brain injury	110
References	111

8. Cellular and molecular changes in animal models of posttraumatic epilepsy

Overview	115
Mossy fiber sprouting	115
Reactive astrocytes	115

Aquaporin-4 dysregulation and mislocalization 117
References **118**

9. **Blood-brain barrier disruption**
   and posttraumatic epilepsy

   Overview 119
   Blood-brain barrier permeability in traumatic brain injury 119
   Edema and posttraumatic epilepsy 127
   Tight junctions and posttraumatic epilepsy 127
   Glial influence on the blood-brain barrier
       and posttraumatic epilepsy 129
   References **133**

10. **Inflammation and posttraumatic epilepsy**

    Overview 137
    Chronic neuroinflammation and seizure susceptibility 137
    Glial cells 138
    Cytokines 141
    References **148**

11. **Biomarkers and treatment trials in animal models**
    to prevent posttraumatic epilepsy

    Overview 153
    Biomarkers 153
    Treatment trials 156
    "Two-hit" injury models 160
    References **165**

12. **Therapeutic targets and future directions**

    Overview 169
    Potential therapeutic targets 169
    Future directions for preclinical posttraumatic epilepsy research 173
    Summary **177**
    References **177**

Index 183

Preface

Posttraumatic epilepsy is a devastating neurological disorder and is a life-long complication of traumatic brain injury. It is a common form of epilepsy and develops in a proportion of traumatic brain injury survivors. There is a critical need for developing new therapeutics and approaches to treat patients with posttraumatic epilepsy, especially since antiepileptic drug prophylaxis is ineffective at preventing the occurrence of late seizures. Much of posttraumatic epilepsy treatment has focused on using antiepileptic drug therapies used to treat other epilepsies. Furthermore, new therapeutic targets are needed since these patients can be refractory to standard antiepileptic drugs.

This book will provide a resource on the history of posttraumatic epilepsy, address our current understanding of the mechanisms of posttraumatic epilepsy, and provide an overview of potential therapeutic targets, while also addressing the many current knowledge gaps. Following an introduction to the history and epidemiology of posttraumatic epilepsy, we consider the neuropathology of posttraumatic epilepsy; clinical trials of antiepileptogenic agents; the role of surgical treatment; and data from animal models including potential mechanisms, biomarkers, and treatment trials.

This book is intended for both scientists and clinicians. Neuroscientists as well as investigators in the fields of epilepsy and traumatic brain injury will find an overview of basic scientific findings and translational studies of posttraumatic epilepsy. Epilepsy researchers who have not fully considered the potential mechanisms responsible for the development of posttraumatic epilepsy will hopefully be stimulated by the book to pursue new, more promising models and unique therapeutic targets for the treatment of posttraumatic epilepsy. Students of all levels, including graduate students, postdoctoral students, and medical students, will learn about posttraumatic epilepsy. Clinicians and clinician-scientists in the field of epilepsy, including neurologists and neurosurgeons involved in the care of patients with posttraumatic epilepsy, will find an abundance of valuable information throughout the book. Translational drug development opportunities, outlined in Chapters 11 and 12, will be of interest to pharmaceutical companies involved in the development of new drugs for posttraumatic epilepsy. We hope this book will serve as a resource for all levels of knowledge-seeking scientists and healthcare and industry professionals. Most importantly, we hope that our book will spark interest in this exciting and emerging field and passion to address and overcome existing treatment gaps in order to improve the lives of patients with traumatic brain injury and posttraumatic epilepsy.

Acknowledgments

I acknowledge my parents (Yolanda, Gilbert, and Gene), my brother (Gilbert H.), and the Jonak family for their unconditional love, support, and encouragement.

I acknowledge my mentors, Djurdjica Coss and Devin Binder, for shaping me into the scientist that I am. Thank you, Devin, for your endless support and inspiration.

Carrie R. Jonak

I acknowledge my parents, Kevin and Jennifer, for their endless love and support. Thank you for supporting all my endeavors in science and in life. Thank you to my father for igniting my interest in STEM at an early age and serving as a role model. Thank you to my mother for teaching me to be strong and to never give up. Thank you both for always believing in me and encouraging me to pursue my dreams!

Allison R. Peterson

I gratefully acknowledge the love and support of my wife Kellie and my children Alexis and Grant, who understand that I navigate several worlds in my career journey.

Devin K. Binder

Chapter 1

History of posttraumatic epilepsy

Overview

Posttraumatic epilepsy (PTE) is a recurrent seizure disorder caused by traumatic brain injury (TBI). In this chapter, we review some historical aspects of PTE. We trace some of the early recognition that head trauma may lead to seizures. Both the conception of epilepsy and its interaction with methods of treatment of TBI evolved from antiquity through medieval and Renaissance practitioners. Key to a more modern and logical approach to diagnosis and treatment of PTE was the emerging understanding of cortical localization beginning in the 1870s. This paralleled the rise of neurology and neurosurgery as localization-based diagnosis and treatment were tested and proven. Despite these advances, however, by the 1920s, the understanding of the neuropathology and pathophysiology of PTE was still in its infancy.

Hippocrates

The words "epilepsy" and "epileptic" are of Greek origin from the root *epilambanein,* which means to seize or to attack. The earliest detailed descriptions of the phenomenology of epilepsy were by the Babylonians in the 2nd millennium BC [1]. It was the Babylonians' perception that seizures resulted from the invasion of the body by a particular evil spirit, which presaged the Greek concept of the "The Sacred Disease" in which the supernatural invasion was by gods [1,2]. Hippocrates (460–370 BC) (Fig. 1.1) was born on the island of Kos, off the Doric coast of what is now Turkey, but studied in Athens and traveled extensively [3]. Hippocrates was the first to identify the brain as the organ associated with epilepsy [4]. This is recorded in the book *On the Sacred Disease* at about the year 400 BC:

> *Mankind must realize that there is but a single organ from which come our pleasures, joys, laughter and wit. From that organ also comes our sorrow, grief, anxiety and lamentation. The brain is in fact that organ; from it comes our intellect, and our vision, and our hearing. Through it we judge the ugly and the beautiful, the noble and the ignoble, the pleasant and the unpleasant…And it is from the brain that we become mad and delirious…Based on the foregoing concepts I believe that the brain is the most powerful organ in man [5,6].*

Posttraumatic Epilepsy. https://doi.org/10.1016/B978-0-323-90099-7.00013-7

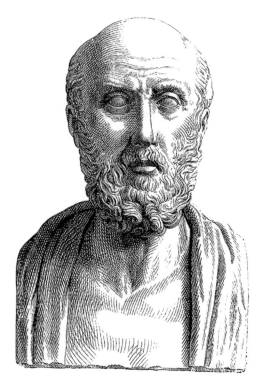

FIG. 1.1 Hippocrates of Kos (460–370 BC). Greek physician of the Age of Pericles (Classical Greece) sometimes termed the "Father of Medicine." The Hippocratic school of medicine revolutionized ancient Greek medicine, establishing medicine as a profession.

On the Sacred Disease comprises the first monograph on epilepsy that we possess. Interestingly, the word "sacred" is ironic in the sense that the message of the book is that epilepsy is instantiated in the brain and is not therefore in that sense more "divine" or "sacred" than any other disease. This conceptualization of epilepsy as arising from the brain and the brain only has therapeutic implications that it can and must be treated not with magical incantations and sorceries but rather by diet, drugs, and (possibly) surgery [4]. According to *On the Sacred Disease*, seizures themselves were caused by stagnation of phlegm but are also influenced by other factors such as the winds [5]. The identity of the author of the book *On the Sacred Disease* is unknown; he is thought to have been one of the anonymous physicians whose writings go under the name "Hippocrates" as part of the *corpus Hippocraticum* (Hippocratic canon, a heterogeneous collection of about 60 medical treatises largely gathered during the Alexandrian era (4th century BC) reflecting the teaching of the school of the Ionic island of Kos [5]).

Writings of the *corpus Hippocraticum* were also the first to clearly describe the extent of experience with head injuries in classical antiquity. The treatise *On Wounds of the Head* is a short surgical text written as a guide to the diagnosis and treatment of head injury [5]. It begins with a detailed description of cranial anatomy, recognizing, for example, that "the bone along the temples is the weakest" [5,7] (modern understanding: the temporal bone is the thinnest cranial bone and most susceptible to traumatic fracture). Next, fractures of the cranium are categorized into six types: (1) fissured fractures; (2) contusion without fracture; (3) depressed fractures; (4) *hedra*, or dents in the skull caused by weapons; (5) cranial lesions away from the scalp wound (*contrecoup* fractures); and (6) wounds above cranial sutures [8]. Finally, each of these fracture types is separately discussed regarding etiology, evaluation, treatment, and prognosis. Interestingly, the treatise mentions little about injury to the brain itself but rather serves as a guide to treatment of skull injuries. However, of key importance to posttraumatic epilepsy and with a hint of early cerebral localization, it is noted that a wound of the left side of the head would cause convulsions on the right side of the body and *vice versa*:

> *And, for the most part, convulsions seize the other side of the body; for, if the wound be situated on the left side, the convulsions will seize the right side of the body; or if the wound be on the right side of the head, the convulsion attacks the left side of the body [7,9].*

The Middle Ages and Renaissance

By the Middle Ages, the term "sacred disease" had been replaced with various versions of the "falling sickness" (*morbus caducus*) [4]. In addition, the conflation of epilepsy with mental disorders became marked during the transition from antiquity to the Middle Ages, with epilepsy now associated with "possession" or "lunacy." The Galenic conception of humors and humors being out of balance in epilepsy was now combined with the medieval idea of demoniac possession. In Temkin's words, "the devil does not cause the epileptic attack by his own power," rather "he exerts his influence when the body is off balance, the humors being stirred up and the brain affected" [4].

Gradually, Renaissance conceptions of humanism led to further observations and further writings on epilepsy and on individual cases. In this context, many of the publications refer to various factors which precede the onset of epileptic attacks. Thus, attention was paid to head injury as a precipitating factor for epilepsy. Valescus de Tharanta (1523) described a head wound in a man that penetrated to the pia mater resulting in accumulation of a "fetid ichor" which caused multiple seizures per day until his death several days later [4,10]. Jacopo Berengario da Carpi (1460–1530) (Fig. 1.2), the son of a barber surgeon [11], published a comprehensive book dealing entirely with head injuries (*De fractura calve sive cranei*) in 1518 [12]. In this treatise, he described six patients who survived severe brain injuries. One case was a man who had seizures 60 days after head injury (hence posttraumatic epilepsy). He placed the man feet up and head down, opened the wound and evacuated copious fluid with the

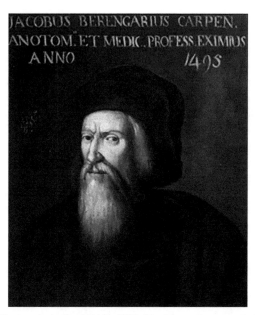

FIG. 1.2 Jacopo Berengario da Carpi (1460–1530). Physician and surgeon. Published *De fractura cranei* in 1518, a landmark work on head injuries (Fig. 1.3). Treated Lorenzo de' Medici, Duke of Urbino, who had been shot in the head in 1517. Also described the anatomy of the meninges, cranial nerves, and ventricular system. *(Reproduced with permission from Parent A. Berengario da Carpi and the renaissance of brain anatomy. Front Neuroanat 2019;13:11.)*

color of milk, after which the epilepsy ceased [13]. The title page of the 3rd edition of his treatise (published in 1535) shows some of the weapons associated with head injuries at the time (Fig. 1.3).

It was also realized that epilepsy may begin many years after head injury (the concept of latency to posttraumatic epilepsy after traumatic brain injury). Ludovicius Duretus (1527–86) reported that:

> *A bone of the skull of a 12-year-old youth had been broken and depressed by a fall and had by negligence not been restored. The brain was therefore hindered in its growth, since the injured bone itself could not grow so as to become able to hold a larger brain. Consequently, in his eighteenth year, the youth suffered from epilepsy because of the oppression of the brain. He was, however, cured by the perforation of the depressed bone, for thus the oppression of the brain was removed [4,14].*

Trephination to craniotomy: Early surgical approaches to epilepsy

Trephination (making a hole in the skull) has been practiced for many centuries [3,15–18]. Trephination is extensively discussed in Hippocrates' *On Wounds in the Head* [8]. One major indication for trephination followed the Galenic

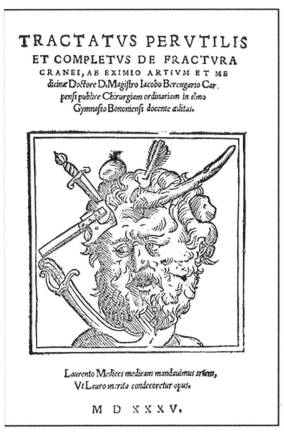

FIG. 1.3 Title page of *De fractura cranei* by Jacopo Berengario da Carpi from 3rd edition (Venice, 1535). First published in Bologna in 1518. Considered the first modern treatise specifically devoted to head injuries. It offered Renaissance surgeons instructions for management of skull fractures and explanations of various surgical instruments and techniques. *(Reproduced with permission from Parent A. Berengario da Carpi and the renaissance of brain anatomy. Front Neuroanat 2019;13:11.)*

conception of humoral imbalance and trephination then allowed evil humors to escape in certain cases [3]. The *Quattuor magistri*, a 13th-century surgical text, recommended opening the skulls of melancholics, epileptics, and others so that the humors and air could be expelled [4]. Such practices persisted over many centuries. In the 17th century, Riverius in *The Compleat Practice of Physick* stated that:

> *If all means fail the last remedy is to open the fore part of the Skull with a Trepan, at distance from the Sutures, that the evil air may breathe out. By this means many times desperate Epilepsies have been cured, and it may be safely done if the Chyurgeon be skillful [19].*

Gradually over time, however, the indications for trephination for epilepsy became limited to: (1) a morbid condition of the skull such as contusion or fracture; and (2) accumulation of humors directly under the skull. The older notion of giving outlet to vapors and humors gradually gave way over time to the concept of treating a localized pathological condition of the brain and its membranes [4].

In the 19th century, trephination continued to be practiced for traumatic epilepsy and diseased bone of the skull. The indication was usually based on the concept of mechanical irritation of the subjacent brain tissue [20]. One key American proponent of this operation was Benjamin Winslow Dudley (1785–1870) [21] (Fig. 1.4).

Dudley was born in Virginia in 1785, and by the next year, his family had moved to Kentucky. He received an M.D. degree from the University of Pennsylvania in 1806 [21,22]. In 1810, he traveled to France and England to study surgery, and in particular became acquainted with trephination in London and Paris [21]. In 1799, Transylvania University had been founded in Lexington, Kentucky, the first school of medicine west of the Allegheny Mountains; and in

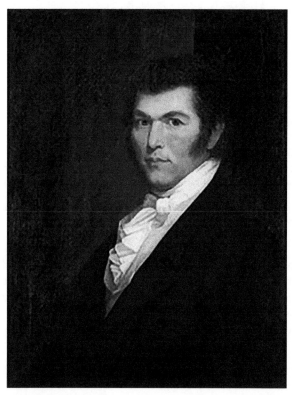

FIG. 1.4 Benjamin Winslow Dudley (1785–1870). Prominent Kentucky surgeon known for trephination for posttraumatic epilepsy.

1817, Dudley was appointed Professor of Surgery and Anatomy at Transylvania University. Between 1819 and 1832, he reported his experiences with trephination for posttraumatic epilepsy in six patients [23,24]. In one case of epilepsy after a gunshot wound to the head, Dudley removed bone fragments resulting in the relief of seizures, and opined that "the brain will bear severe mechanical irritation for a great length of time, without fatal disorganization and that the use of the trephine under such circumstances may restore the organ to its former healthy condition" [24]. This was the largest recorded series of such cases to date, and it stimulated other American surgeons to consider trephination for posttraumatic epilepsy. The stated rationale for trephination in these cases was to remove the cause of "cerebral excitement" and restore "corporeal and intellectual function" [21].

Following Dudley's experience, in 1852, Stephen Smith published a survey of 27 trephination cases performed in the United States between 1819 and 1850 [25]. While indicating its effectiveness in individual cases in which a proper indication existed, he did cautiously note the "unjustifiable haste of surgeons in reporting their cases, before sufficient time has elapsed after the operation to give a rational opinion as to its success" [25]. Similar observations were made by John Shaw Billings who reviewed 72 cases (not all from the United States) performed between 1806 and 1860 [26]. In 1884, W.T. Briggs of Tennessee, a student of Dudley, reported 30 cases of posttraumatic epilepsy operated to relieve "accentuated pressure upon the membrane of the brain [dura] from fractures of the skull" [27]. Over the last decades of the 19th century, other trephination series were reported; in general, the "cure" rate decreased due to longer follow-up, but the death rate also decreased probably due to greater use of antiseptic techniques (introduced after Lister and Pasteur) [28].

Early pioneers in cortical localization

Since antiquity, trephination had been based on either a nonanatomic "release" of humors from the brain more diffusely or obvious external pathology to guide location of trephination (such as Dudley's treatment of a gunshot wound to the brain). What were the developments that subsequently allowed more logical interpretation of localization of pathology causing seizures? In the latter half of the 19th century, early pioneers in cortical localization made critical discoveries enabling subsequent localization-based diagnosis and treatment.

Localization of language functions

Paul Broca (Fig. 1.5) was born in the Bordeaux area of France in 1824, the son of a former surgeon in Napoleon's service. He attended medical school in Paris. Ultimately, he became a "Prosector" performing anatomic dissections for medical lectures at the University of Paris and later was appointed to positions in pathology and surgery. Interestingly, he accepted Charles Darwin's theory of evolution by natural selection (*On the Origin of Species* was published in 1859)

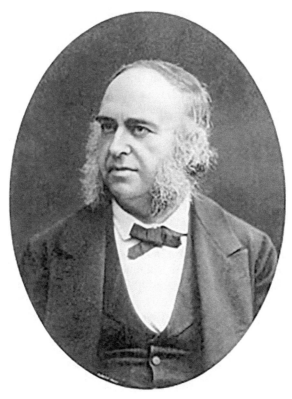

FIG. 1.5 Pierre Paul Broca (1824–80). French physician, anatomist, and anthropologist. Best known for research on the eponymous "Broca's area," a region of the dominant frontal lobe critical for expressive language function. Broca also contributed to the science of anthropometry and physical anthropology.

and once remarked, "I would rather be a transformed ape than a degenerate son of Adam" [29]. Ironically perhaps, Broca died of a brain hemorrhage in 1880 at the age of 56.

While Broca also contributed significantly to the field of anthropometry and physical anthropology, including founding the *Société d'Anthropologie de Paris* (1859) and the journal *Revue d'Anthropologie* (1872), it was his discovery of the speech production center of the brain that was profoundly important to modern neurology and neurosurgery. In 1861, Broca visited Louis Victor Leborgne, a patient in the Bicêtre Hospital whose case was distinguished by intact comprehension but the inability to speak any words other than "tan" (hence, thereafter, Mr. Leborgne has ever been known as "Tan" to the scientific community) [3,30]. At autopsy, Broca found a "chronic and progressive softening" in the third frontal convolution of the left hemisphere (in a location we would now call the left inferior frontal gyrus, adjacent to the Sylvian fissure). Broca collected more cases with autopsy evidence of left frontal lesion localization and published these cases in 1865 as *On the Site of the Faculty of Articulated Speech* [31,32]. In that publication, Broca confidently stated "Nous parlon avec l'hemisphere gauche" ("we speak with the left hemisphere"). These cases as well as Broca's authority convinced the scientific and clinical world for the first time that the cortical locality of expressive language (Broca's area) had been discovered. Miraculously, Leborgne's brain survived wars and neglect in museum basements and was rediscovered in the late 1970s and subjected to CT scans which confirmed damage confined to Broca's area [33] (Fig. 1.6).

"Broca's aphasia" came to connote expressive aphasia characterized by impairment in speech output with intact comprehension, which is distinguished from "Wernicke's aphasia" named for Carl Wernicke (1848–1905) (also termed "receptive" aphasia) characterized by impairment in language comprehension. Carl Wernicke (Fig. 1.7) was a German physician and neuropathologist who was directly influenced by Broca's findings. In 1874, just 9 years after Broca's 1865 publication, Wernicke published *Der Aphasische Symptomencomplex* [34], which described sensory (receptive or Wernicke's) aphasia as distinct from motor (expressive or Broca's) aphasia, and demonstrated its cause by lesions of the left *temporal* lobe (specifically the posterior superior temporal gyrus). Thus, by the mid-1870s, the foundation for the neuroanatomical bases for both expressive and receptive language had been established.

Localization of motor functions

Meanwhile, other investigators would localize motor functions in the brain. Gustav Fritsch (Fig. 1.8) was an anatomist and physiologist who studied natural science and medicine and in addition to his studies of the brain was also involved with ethnographical research in southern Africa, archaeology and zoology. Eduard Hitzig (Fig. 1.9) was a neurologist and neuropsychiatrist who studied medicine at the Universities of Berlin and Würzburg. In 1870, Fritsch

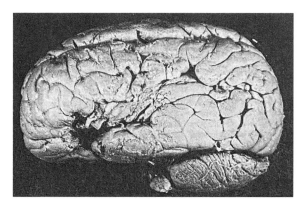

FIG. 1.6 The brain of Leborgne (nicknamed "Tan"). *(Reproduced with permission from Finger S, Minds behind the brain: a history of the pioneers and their discoveries. Oxford: Oxford University Press; 2000.)*

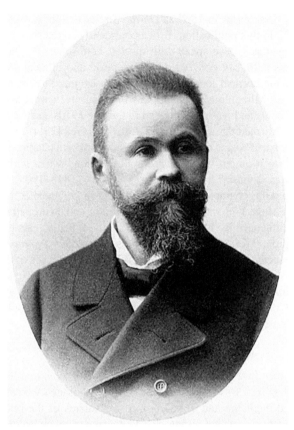

FIG. 1.7 Carl Wernicke (1848–1905). German physician and neuropathologist. Best known for research on the eponymous "Wernicke's area," a region of the dominant temporal lobe critical for receptive language function.

and Hitzig applied electrical stimulation to the exposed cerebral cortex of a dog without anesthesia. These experiments were reportedly performed on a dressing table in a bedroom of Hitzig's house in Berlin [3]. They found that stimulation of specific areas caused involuntary muscle contractions of parts of the dog's body. They identified and mapped the brain's "motor strip" in the frontal lobe (what we now call precentral gyrus). These experiments represented the discovery of the motor cortex, and were published in 1870 [35].

David Ferrier (Fig. 1.10) was born in 1843 in Aberdeen, Scotland, trained in medicine at the University of Edinburgh, and then moved to London and was appointed as a neuropathologist in 1871. Importantly, Ferrier worked at the same hospital (National Hospital for Paralysis and Epilepsy, Queen Square) as the neurologist John Hughlings Jackson (see below). Ferrier was greatly influenced by Hughlings Jackson, who was aiming to localize brain functions on clinical grounds. Ferrier and Hughlings Jackson often joined neurological

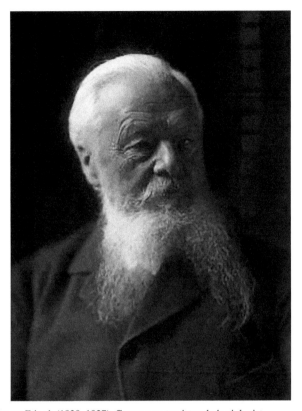

FIG. 1.8   Gustav Fritsch (1838–1927). German anatomist and physiologist.

meetings organized by the psychiatrist James Crichton-Browne (1840–1938), one of Ferrier's classmates at Edinburgh, at the West Riding Lunatic Asylum in Yorkshire. Together, they discussed the experiments of Fritsch and Hitzig. Ferrier embarked on experiments to extend Fritsch and Hitzig's findings of electrical stimulation of the motor cortex in dogs to other species [36]. Using low-intensity faradic stimulation of the cortex in multiple species including dogs, birds, guinea pigs, rabbits, and later macaque monkeys [37], Ferrier was able to produce detailed maps of motor functions [3]. Ferrier also lesioned the areas to demonstrate loss of specific motor functions [3]. He published two notable books (*The Functions of the Brain*, 1876, and *The Localization of Brain Disease*, 1878), which summarized his experimental results and explicitly applied them to clinical applications of cortical localization. Together with Hughlings Jackson and Crichton-Browne, Ferrier co-founded the journal *Brain* in 1878; and together with Hughlings Jackson and the neurologist William Gowers co-founded the National Society for the Employment of Epileptics in 1892 (still extant in the United Kingdom as the National Society for Epilepsy, a medical charity for people with epilepsy).

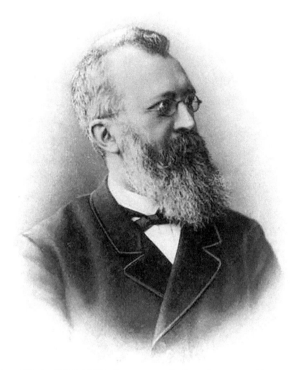

FIG. 1.9   Eduard Hitzig (1838–1907). German neurologist and neuropsychiatrist.

Thus, by the mid-1870s, these early pioneers in cortical localization had laid the foundation for localization-induced functions in the brain (both language and motor functions). These findings would provide critical experimental support to the clinical deductions of John Hughlings Jackson and the other neurologists and neurosurgeons who followed.

Rise of neurology and neurosurgery in parallel in the 1870s and 1880s

John Hughlings Jackson

John Hughlings Jackson (1835–1911) (Fig. 1.11), often considered the father of British neurology, is credited with laying the foundations of modern understanding of epilepsy. He was born in 1835 at Providence Green near Harrogate, Yorkshire, and ultimately attended the York Medical and Surgical School. In 1862, he was appointed Assistant Physician at the recently founded National Hospital for Paralysis and Epilepsy in Queen Square, and he set out to improve neurological nosology (diagnostic categorization). Hughlings Jackson's studies of unilateral convulsions are immortalized in the eponym "Jacksonian epilepsy" [38] and in particular he was interested in the "march" of the seizure over the body

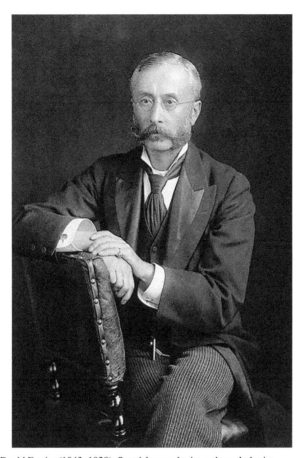

FIG. 1.10   David Ferrier (1843–1928). Scottish neurologist and psychologist.

parts. This "Jacksonian march" implied somatotopic organization, and based on clinical evidence Hughlings Jackson surmised the presence of a somatotopically organized motor cortex. Hughlings Jackson's genius throughout his career was his ability to extract general principles of brain organization and anatomic localization based on detailed clinical observations and autopsies. Of course, by the early 1870s, the experimental investigations of Fritsch and Hitzig and then Ferrier (see above) regarding cortical localization lent experimental support to Hughlings Jackson's clinical deductions [39–41]. Indeed, in 1900 Hitzig stated in retrospect that his physiological experiments only confirmed the conclusions that Hughlings Jackson had reached by deduction from clinical observations [39].

Jacksonian (focal motor) seizures also informed Hughlings Jackson's evolving concept of the nature of epilepsy. By 1873, in a famous article, he defined epilepsy as "occasional, sudden, excessive, rapid, and local discharges of gray matter" [42].

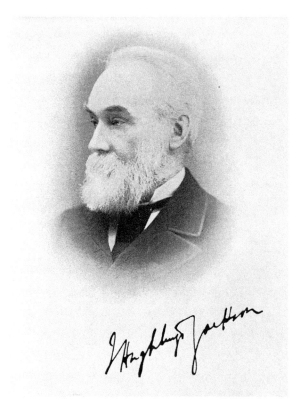

FIG. 1.11 John Hughlings Jackson (1835–1911). Pioneering English neurologist often considered the "father of British neurology" known for diagnosis and understanding of epilepsy. Among many important findings, he described the concept of a "discharging" lesion as etiologic in cases of focal epilepsy, the "Jacksonian" march of symptoms in focal motor seizures, and the so-called dreamy state in psychomotor seizures of temporal lobe origin.

Most critical to the pathologic underpinnings of posttraumatic epilepsy would prove to be Hughlings Jackson's enduring concept that focal injury to the brain creates a "discharging lesion" from which seizures could subsequently arise. In particular, Hughlings Jackson's theoretical physiological approach that epileptic convulsions involved excessive but also *local* discharges of gray matter reinforced the idea that epilepsy was symptomatic of local brain pathology such as vascular lesions, tumors, or scars [2]. This would later stimulate Wilder Penfield's desire to search for the cellular substrate in the brain of Hughlings Jackson's "discharging lesion" [43,44] (Chapter 3).

Victor Horsley and William McEwen

On August 13, 1886, the surgeon Victor Horsley (Fig. 1.12), then a 29-year-old recruit to the burgeoning National Hospital for Paralysis and Epilepsy in Queen Square, addressed the Section on Surgery of the British Medical Association

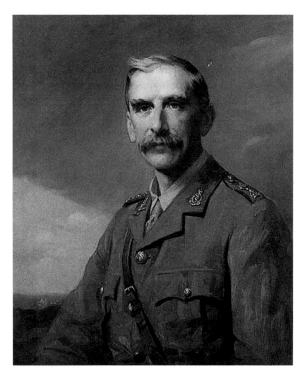

FIG. 1.12   Victor Horsley (1857–1916). English surgeon and physiologist. Developed many practical neurosurgical techniques including hemostatic bone wax, the skin flap, the transcranial approach to the pituitary gland, the division of the trigeminal nerve root to treat trigeminal neuralgia, and the first stereotactic device (Horsley-Clarke apparatus developed with Robert H. Clarke in 1908). As a neuroscientist, carried out studies with faradic electrical stimulation of the brain. Along with William MacEwen, was the first to explore intraoperative electrical stimulation of the cortex for the localization of epileptic foci in humans.

on "Advances in the Surgery of the Central Nervous System." He presented three successful brain operations at the National Hospital on patients with epilepsy [45,46]. Two cases were caused by trauma and one case by tumor. Horsley mentioned the work in monkeys that had made the correct diagnosis possible. Both the French neurologist Jean-Martin Charcot (1825–1893) and Hughlings Jackson attended his presentation, and "Dr. Hughlings Jackson warmly congratulated Mr. Victor Horsley on the success of his operations on the brain." The manuscript was published that year in the *British Medical Journal* [46]. This manuscript was subsequently considered to have inaugurated the modern era of surgical therapy for epilepsy [47]. The very next year, in 1887, Horsley reported a series of 10 cases including cases in which he used faradic stimulation to localize cortical areas [48]. For example, case #5: "October 19th, 1886. Trephining over 'facial centre,' and removal of cortex composing that centre as determined by faradism at the time" [48]. It is intriguing that Horsley's first faradic stimulation in humans came directly after his collaboration with the physiologist Edward Schäfer (1850–1935) [49] and the neurologist Charles Beevor (1854–1908) [50] with faradic stimulation experiments in monkeys confirming and extending Ferrier's research [4]. Soon, other surgeons such as the celebrated American neurosurgeon William Keen (1837–1932) [51] adopted these techniques [52].

In 1888, the Scottish surgeon William MacEwen (Fig. 1.13), who was well acquainted with the work of Jackson and Ferrier, addressed the same society and reported on his pioneering work in brain surgery, much of which antedated Horsley's [4]. His manuscript was also published that year in the *British Medical Journal* [53]. One case he reported was that of a convulsion accompanied by loss of consciousness and postictal right hemiplegia and aphasia of two hours' duration. (Postictal paralysis of the contralateral limbs was originally

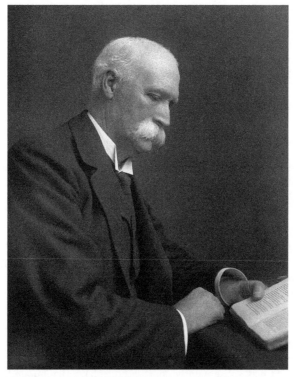

FIG. 1.13 William MacEwen (1848–1924). Scottish surgeon who applied the work of Jackson and Ferrier to become the first to demonstrate successful intracranial surgery where the site of the lesion was localized solely by preoperative focal epileptic signs. Made multiple other contributions to medicine immortalized in part by several eponyms: *MacEwen's triangle* (a surgical landmark on the surface of the temporal bone just superior to the external auditory canal used to locate the level of the mastoid antrum), *MacEwen's operation* (for inguinal hernia), and *MacEwen's sign* (for hydrocephalus and brain abscess).

described by Robert Bentley Todd (1809–60) and subsequently came to be called "Todd's paralysis" and has served as a localizing sign for seizure onset location ever since [54].) Based on the postictal right hemiplegia and aphasia, MacEwen diagnosed an abscess "in the immediate vicinity of Broca's lobe" and, while he was not given permission to perform the operation with the patient alive, after the patient's death the procedure was performed and the abscess was found exactly in the location as diagnosed. This shows an early localization of a cerebral lesion simply based on neurological signs and also prompted MacEwen to lament that this finding "gave poignancy to the regret that the operation had not been permitted during life" [53].

MacEwen was likely the first to surgically excise a cortical "discharging lesion" in 1879. In a case reported in 1888 [53], in 1879, he operated on a patient at the Royal Infirmary in Glasgow who had seizures arising from the right face and arm leading McEwen to surmise that there was evidence of an "irritation to the lower and middle portions of the ascending convolutions…in the left frontal lobe" [53]. McEwen trephined the patient on the left side and a dural tumor was found spreading over the left frontal lobe which was removed. When the patient died 8 years later from glomerulonephritis ("Bright's disease"), autopsy found no trace of residual or recurrent tumor. This case provides the first example of surgical intervention based solely on the anatomical relationship between the "discharging lesion" and clinical manifestations of the seizures, vindicating the clinical and physiological rationale of Hughlings Jackson a decade earlier [42]. MacEwen was so impressed by the advantage of using the new maps of the cortex to localize surgical pathology that he subsequently operated on several more cases [3,55].

Toward the 20th century and localization-related epilepsy

By the end of the 19th century, with the modern concept of localization-related epilepsy taking form with the observations of Hughlings Jackson and cerebral localization of language by Broca and Wernicke and motor functions by Fritsch, Hitzig, and Ferrier translating into human brain mapping with the work of Horsley and McEwen, focal structural lesions of the brain could for the first time be deduced based on anatomic principles and/or mapped *in situ*. Such groundwork would lead eventually to the detailed intraoperative cortical mapping pioneered by Wilder Penfield [44]. However, the optimism afforded by this new anatomic understanding together with modern antisepsis perhaps led to overreach in the application of trephination/craniotomy after head trauma. In 1891, the prominent Philadelphia surgeon David Agnew (1818–92) opined that "Whenever the profession can accept the doctrine that all depressed fractures, however slight…and entirely irrespective of pressure symptoms, are proper subjects for trephining, then will traumatic epilepsy largely disappear from the list of surgical diseases" [56]. Agnew's hyperbole was dialed back by other practitioners as more experience was gained [28]. In particular, William Keen himself together with his colleague W. Taylor, Attending Surgeon to the Orthopedics Hospital and Infirmary for Nervous Disease, Philadelphia, stated:

> *For a time we [the author and Dr. Keen] hit almost every head [of patients with epilepsy] that came our way...At first, ...the purely surgical results, the carpenter work, ...were brilliant, so brilliant in fact that we became enthusiastic and believed that in surgery the long looked for treatment of epilepsy had been found. As our experience ripened and sufficient time elapsed for us to see the real neurological results our enthusiasm waned, our disappointments were many, and finally we were compelled to modify our opinion and confine this method of treatment to a very limited number of carefully selected cases [57].*

Similarly, not all practitioners of the time fully embraced all of Horsley's ideas for epilepsy surgery [58]. Moses Allen Starr (1854–1932) (Fig. 1.14), pioneering American neurologist and Professor of Diseases of the Mind and the Nervous System at Columbia College, New York, published a book *Brain*

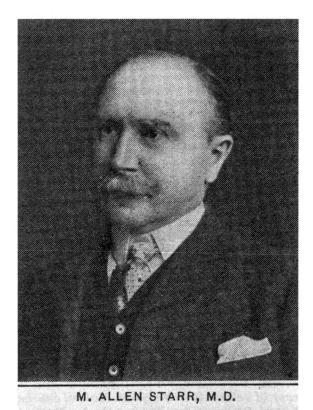

M. ALLEN STARR, M.D.

FIG. 1.14 Moses Allen Starr (1854–1932). Internationally famous American neurologist in New York. Was President of the New York Neurological Society and also President of the American Neurological Association.

Surgery in 1893 summarizing the status of brain surgery at the time [59]. In the book, he discussed traumatic epilepsy and in particular reported detailed clinical study of 13 patients operated by his New York colleague Dr. Charles McBurney for seizures after head injury, usually due to fracture or skull defect [59]. Of these cases, Starr reported "cured 3; improved 5; not improved 4; died 1" [59]. He also reviewed other contemporary cases in the literature. Interestingly, Starr (*contra* Horsley) did not think that excising injured cortex would be beneficial for seizure reduction as doing so would be followed by formation of a scar (cicatrix) that itself would give rise to localized epilepsy. He referred to two of Horsley's cases that had recurrent seizures despite cortical excision. He concluded that, while "some patients have undoubtedly been cured," "in the majority there has been failure to permanently cure epilepsy by operative interference" [59].

Fedor Krause

Fedor Krause (1857–1937) (Fig. 1.15) was the next influential neurosurgeon to become experienced in the surgical treatment of epilepsy [58,60–62]. Krause was born in Friedland in Lower Silesia (today Mieroszów in Poland), and his family moved to Berlin when he was 9 years old [60]. Krause originally studied music at the Conservatory of Music in Berlin and was considered a piano virtuoso but then switched to medicine and graduated from Friedrich Wilhelm University (since 1949 called Humboldt University) in Berlin. Between 1893 and 1912, he operated on 96 patients for the treatment of epilepsy [58]. Many of his operations were done using faradic current stimulation of the exposed motor cortex; in so doing, Krause produced the first accurate maps of the human motor strip [63] (Fig. 1.16). "I had the good fortune to be in a position to faradically irritate the human 'motor area' during a great number of surgical operations on the brain" [63]. Krause recognized that focal epilepsy could be due to a cortical scar, and he focused in particular on posttraumatic scarring as an etiology for focal epilepsy [64,65]. Of importance, Krause also recognized that the brain area responsible for seizures (what Hughlings Jackson called the "discharging lesion" and what modern epileptology terms the "epileptogenic zone") may be more extensive than the actual structural lesion found at operation. Regarding Starr's objection that operating just creates another cicatrix and recurrent seizures, Krause held that "the objection brought forward that after such excisions, the scar will recur during the process of healing, has no foundation…our experiences teach us that scars resulting from aseptic operations will, in themselves, not give rise to irritations or epilepsy" [65]. Krause also made other contributions to neurosurgery, such as the monumental contribution *Surgery of the Brain and Spinal Cord* encompassing all of contemporary neurosurgery (published first in Germany 1908–11) [63] and the technical development of specific neurosurgical procedures which have come to be called the "Krause operations" [60,66]. Krause ceased his surgical practice in 1930 and settled in Rome to devote himself to music and fine arts, passing away in 1937 [60].

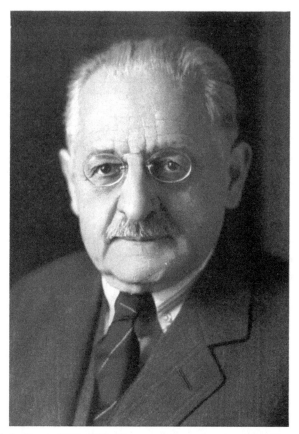

FIG. 1.15   Fedor Krause (1857–1937). German neurosurgeon and musician. First to make accurate maps of the human motor strip. Contributed significant experience in surgery for posttraumatic epilepsy. Published the monumental treatise *Surgery of the Brain and Spinal Cord* encompassing all of contemporary neurosurgery (published first in Germany 1908–11). Responsible for the technical development of specific neurosurgical procedures which have come to be called the "Krause operations." *(Reproduced with permission from Bacigaluppi S, Bragazzi N, Martini M. Fedor Krause (1857–1937): the father of neurosurgery, Neurosurg Rev 2020;43(6):1443–1449.)*

Otfrid Foerster

Otfrid Foerster (1873–1941) (Fig. 1.17) was born in Breslau, a city in Lower Silesia which at the time was Prussian but is now Wrocław in Poland (Fig. 1.18) [58,67–69]. He studied medicine in Freiburg, Kiel, and Breslau and then studied abroad in France and Switzerland. Foerster was actually a neurologist trained by J. Jules Dejerine (1849–1917) and Carl Wernicke (1848–1905) prior to taking up the scalpel himself as a surgeon. Together, Wernicke (see above) and Foerster published a brain atlas (*Atlas des Gehirns*) in 1903 [70].

Like Krause, Foerster performed cortical stimulation under local anesthesia before resection of epileptogenic areas [58,71]. In 1924, he was the first

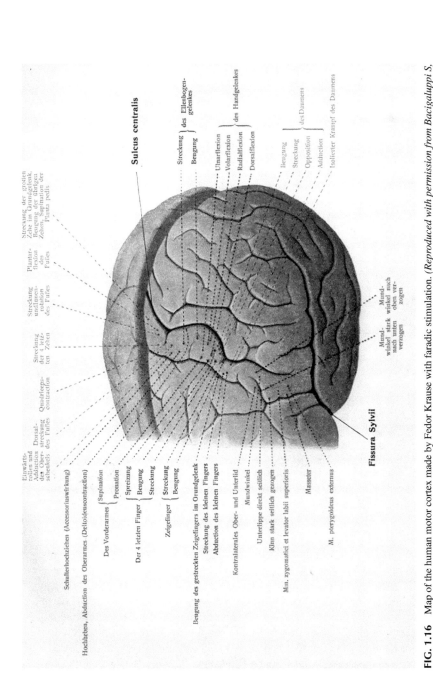

FIG. 1.16 Map of the human motor cortex made by Fedor Krause with faradic stimulation. *(Reproduced with permission from Bacigaluppi S, Bragazzi N, Martini M. Fedor Krause (1857–1937): the father of neurosurgery. Neurosurg Rev 2020;43(6):1443–1449.)*

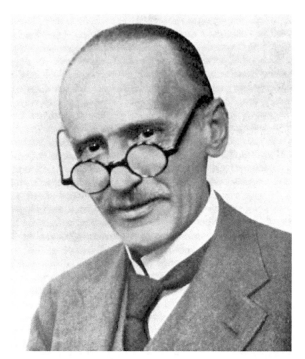

FIG. 1.17   Otfrid Foerster (1873–1941). German neurologist and neurosurgeon. Made many contributions to neurology and neurosurgery, including description of the dermatomes, motor cortex mapping, rhizotomy for the treatment of spasticity, anterolateral cordotomy for pain, Foerster's syndrome, and epilepsy surgery [67]. Also traveled to Russia to treat Lenin after his stroke [62,67]. *(Reproduced with permission from Karenberg A, et al. Historical review: a short history of German neurology—from its origins to the 1940s. Neurol Res Pract 2019;1:14.)*

to report on the use of forced hyperventilation to precipitate a seizure [58]. In 1925, he was the first to apply pneumoencephalography to localize the cicatricial (scarred) area in patients with posttraumatic epilepsy [71]. Later, he was also the first to use intraoperative electrocorticography (reported in 1935) [72] following the description of the human electroencephalogram (EEG) by Hans Berger in 1929 [73].

For posttraumatic epilepsy in particular, Foerster promoted radical excision of the scarred cortex down to the ventricle in posttraumatic epileptic patients. The idea was that reducing mechanical traction from the scar would reduce the irritation of the cortex and hence the seizure frequency [74]. Analysis of resected specimens from these cases with his collaborator Wilder Penfield led to the first pathological studies of posttraumatic epilepsy (Chapter 3) [74].

As for Krause, it is clear that Foerster's localization-minded clinical practice owed much to the example set forth by Hughlings Jackson. By 1936, at the end of his career, Foerster stated: "The map of the human motor cortex to be found nowadays in every textbook of neurology is nothing else but a copy of the picture engraved in Hughlings Jackson's brain" [75].

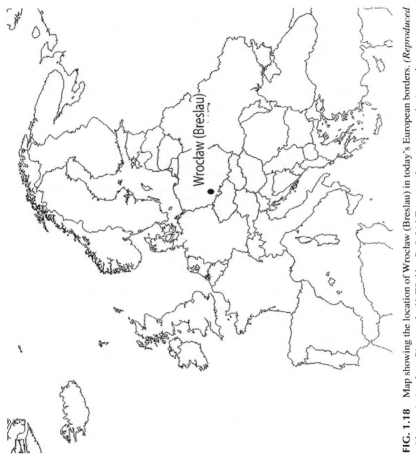

FIG. 1.18 Map showing the location of Wrocław (Breslau) in today's European borders. (*Reproduced with permission from Piotrowska N, Winkler P, Offrid Foerster, the great neurologist and neurosurgeon from Breslau (Wrocław): his influence on early neurosurgeons and legacy to present-day neurosurgery. J Neurosurg 2007;107(2):451–456.*)

Thus, by the early 1920s, the pioneering work of Hughlings Jackson with ample experimental support as described above had clearly developed and entrenched the localizationist trend in clinical neurology. Pioneering neurosurgeons (such as Horsley, MacEwen, Krause, and Foerster) practiced applied neurology to localize lesions for surgical extirpation. However, at that time (~ 1 century ago now), there were still many unknowns. First, the epidemiology of PTE was unclear, despite oblique references, for example, to a proportion of Franco-Prussian War casualties developing PTE [59]. Twentieth-century wars would provide ample data in this regard (Chapter 2). Second, the neuropathology of PTE had not yet been studied with modern histological techniques developed by Golgi, Cajal, and Río-Hortega (Chapter 3). Third, imaging was in its infancy (far removed from the ability of modern computerized tomography (CT) and magnetic resonance imaging (MRI) to noninvasively define pathology). Fourth, there remained little to no understanding of the pathophysiology of posttraumatic epilepsy. The latter is the topic of much of the rest of this book!

References

[1] Reynolds EH, Kinnier Wilson JV. Psychoses of epilepsy in Babylon: the oldest account of the disorder. Epilepsia 2008;49(9):1488–90.

[2] Reynolds EH, Rodin E. The clinical concept of epilepsy. Epilepsia 2009;50(Suppl 3):2–7.

[3] Finger S. Origins of neuroscience: a history of explorations into brain function. New York, NY: Oxford University Press; 1994.

[4] Temkin O. The falling sickness: a history of epilepsy from the Greeks to the beginnings of modern neurology. Baltimore, MD: Johns Hopkins Press; 1971.

[5] Walshe TM. Neurological concepts in ancient Greek medicine. New York: Oxford University Press; 2016.

[6] Hippocrates. On the sacred disease.

[7] Hippocrates. On wounds of the head.

[8] Panourias IG, et al. Hippocrates: a pioneer in the treatment of head injuries. Neurosurgery 2005;57(1):181–9.

[9] Finger S. Minds behind the brain: a history of the pioneers and their discoveries. Oxford: Oxford University Press; 2000.

[10] de Tharanta V. Philonium; 1523. Venice.

[11] Parent A. Berengario da Carpi and the renaissance of brain anatomy. Front Neuroanat 2019;13:11.

[12] Di Ieva A, et al. Berengario da Carpi: a pioneer in neurotraumatology. J Neurosurg 2011;114(5):1461–70.

[13] da Carpi B. De fractura calve sive cranei; 1518. Bologna.

[14] Hollerius J. Omnia opera practica. Doctissimis eiusdem scholiis et observationibus illustrata: Deinde Lud. Dureti in eundem enarrationibus, annotationibus, et Antonii Valetii D. Medici exercitationibus luculentis; 1623. Geneva.

[15] Parry TW. An address on trephination of the living human skull in prehistoric times. Br Med J 1923;1(3246):457–60.

[16] Sturgeon JF. Trephination in the history of medicine. Appl Ther 1962;4:294–302.

[17] Gross CG. A hole in the head: more tales in the history of neuroscience. Cambridge, MA: MIT Press; 2012.

[18] Trelles JO. Cranial trepanation in ancient Peru. World Neurol 1962;3:538–45.

[19] Riverius L. The compleat practice of physick; 1655. London.

[20] Echeverria JG. De la trépanation dans l'épilepsie par traumatismes du crâne. Arch Gen Med 1878;2:529–54. 652-676.

[21] Jensen RL, Stone JL. Benjamin Winslow Dudley and early American trephination for post-traumatic epilepsy. Neurosurgery 1997;41(1):263–8.

[22] Patchell RA, Young AB, Tibbs PA. Benjamin Winslow Dudley and the surgical treatment of epilepsy. Neurology 1987;37(2):290–1.

[23] Dudley BW. Observations on injuries of the head. Transylvania J Med 1828;1:9–40.

[24] Dudley BW. The use of the trephine in epilepsy. Transylvania J Med 1832;5:132–3.

[25] Smith S. The surgical treatment of epilepsy, with statistical tables, comprising all the recorded cases of ligature of the carotid artery: and also of trephining the cranium by American surgeons. N Y J Med 1852;8:220–42.

[26] Billings JS. The surgical treatment of epilepsy. Cincinnati Lancet & Observer 1861;4:334–41.

[27] Briggs WT. The surgical treatment of epilepsy arising from injuries of the head, with special reference to the use of the trephine. Trans Am Surg Assoc 1884;2:101–24.

[28] Friedlander WJ. The history of modern epilepsy: the beginning, 1865–1914. Westport, CT: Greenwood Press; 2001.

[29] Sagan C. Broca's brain. New York, NY: Random House; 1979.

[30] Mohammed N, et al. Louis Victor Leborgne ("Tan"). World Neurosurg 2018;114:121–5.

[31] Broca P. Sur le siège de la faculté du langage articulé. Bull Soc Anthropol 1865;6:337–93.

[32] Berker EA, Berker AH, Smith A. Translation of Broca's 1865 report. Localization of speech in the third left frontal convolution. Arch Neurol 1986;43(10):1065–72.

[33] Signoret JL, et al. Rediscovery of Leborgne's brain: anatomical description with CT scan. Brain Lang 1984;22(2):303–19.

[34] Wernicke C. *Der* Aphasische Symptomencomplex: eine psychologische Studie auf anatomischer basis. Breslau: M. Crohn und Weigert; 1874.

[35] Fritsch G, Hitzig E. Über die elektrische Erregbarkeit des Grosshirns. Arch Anat Pathol 1870;3:300–32.

[36] Greenblatt SH. Cerebral localization: From theory to practice. In: A history of neurosurgery in its scientific and professional contexts. Park Ridge, IL: American Association of Neurological Surgeons; 1997. p. 137–52.

[37] Sandrone S, Zanin E. David Ferrier (1843-1928). J Neurol 2014;261(6):1247–8.

[38] York GK, Koehler PJ. Jacksonian epilepsy. In: Koehler PJ, Bruyn GW, Pearce JMS, editors. Neurological eponyms. New York: Oxford University Press; 2000. p. 94–9.

[39] Hitzig E. Hughlings Jackson and the cortical motor centres in the light of physiological research. Brain 1900;23:545–81.

[40] Jackson JH. On convulsive seizures. Lancet 1890;**1**:685–8. 735–738, 785–788.

[41] Reynolds EH. Todd, Hughlings Jackson, and the electrical basis of epilepsy. Lancet 2001;358:575–7.

[42] Jackson JH. On the anatomical, physiological and pathological investigation of epilepsies. In: West Riding Lunatic Asylum Medical Reports, 3; 1873. p. 315–39.

[43] Penfield W. Introduction (symposium on post-traumatic epilepsy). Epilepsia 1961;2:109–10.

[44] Penfield W. No man alone: a neurosurgeon's life. Boston, MA: Little, Brown and Company; 1977.

[45] Uff C, et al. Sir Victor Horsley's 19th century operations at the National Hospital for Neurology and Neurosurgery, Queen Square. J Neurosurg 2011;114(2):534–42.

[46] Horsley V. Brain-surgery. Br Med J 1886;2:670–5.

[47] Engel J. Surgical treatment of the epilepsies. New York: Raven Press; 1987.

[48] Horsley V. Remarks on ten consecutive cases of operations upon the brain and cranial cavity to illustrate the details and safety of the method employed. Br Med J 1887;1:863–5.

[49] Horsley V, Schäfer EA. A record of experiments upon the functions of the cerebral cortex. Philos Trans R Soc Lond 1888;179:1–45.

[50] Beevor CE, Horsley V. A minute analysis (experimental) of the various movements produced by stimluating in the monkey different regions of the cortical Centre for the upper limb, as defined by Professor Ferrier. Philos Trans R Soc Lond 1888;178:153–67.

[51] Bingham WF, W. W. Keen and the dawn of American neurosurgery. J Neurosurg 1986;64(5):705–12.

[52] Keen WW. Three successful cases of cerebral surgery, including (1) the removal of a large intracranial fibroma; (2) exsection of damaged brain tissue; and (3) exsection of the cerebral Centre for the left hand, with remarks on the general technique of such operations. Trans Am Surg Assoc 1888;6:293–347.

[53] McEwen W. An address on the surgery of the brain and spinal cord. Br Med J 1888;2:302–9.

[54] Binder DK. A history of Todd and his paralysis. Neurosurgery 2004;54(2):480–6.

[55] Walker AE, Green RE. A history of neurological surgery. Baltimore, MD: The Williams & Wilkins Company; 1951.

[56] Agnew D. Present status of brain surgery, based on the practice of Philadelphia surgeons. Boston Med Surg J 1891;125:356–8.

[57] Taylor WJ. The surgical treatment of epilepsy. Trans Coll Phys Phila 1912;34:79–81.

[58] Feindel W, Leblanc R, Villemure J-G. History of the surgical treatment of epilepsy. In: Greenblatt SH, Dagi TF, Epstein MH, editors. A history of neurosurgery in its scientific and professional contexts. Park Ridge, IL: American Association of Neurological Surgeons; 1997.

[59] Starr MA. Brain surgery. New York, NY: William Wood; 1893.

[60] Bacigaluppi S, Bragazzi NL, Martini M. Fedor Krause (1857-1937): the father of neurosurgery. Neurosurg Rev 2020;43(6):1443–9.

[61] Laios K, et al. Fedor Krause (1857-1937) and his innovations in neurosurgery. Surg Innov 2019;26(5):633–5.

[62] Buchfelder M. From trephination to tailored resection: neurosurgery in Germany before World War II. Neurosurgery 2005;56(3):605–13.

[63] Krause F. Die Chirurgie des Gehirns und Rückenmarks nach eigenen Erfahrungen. Berlin und Wien: Urban und Schwarzenberg; 1908-1911.

[64] Krause F. Die Operative Behandlung der Epilepsie. Med Klin Berlin 1909;5:1418–22.

[65] Krause F. Surgery of the brain and spinal cord based on personal experience. (translated by A. Haubold and M. Thorek). New York, NY: Rebman; 1912.

[66] Rosegay H. The Krause operations. J Neurosurg 1992;76(6):1032–6.

[67] Piotrowska N, Winkler PA. Otfrid Foerster, the great neurologist and neurosurgeon from Breslau (Wrocław): his influence on early neurosurgeons and legacy to present-day neurosurgery. J Neurosurg 2007;107(2):451–6.

[68] Tan TC, Black PM. The contributions of Otfrid Foerster (1873-1941) to neurology and neurosurgery. Neurosurgery 2001;49(5):1231–5 [discussion 1235-6].

[69] Karenberg A, et al. Historical review: a short history of German neurology—from its origins to the 1940s. Neurol Res Pract 2019;1:14.

[70] Wernicke C, Foerster O. Atlas des Gehirns. Breslau: Verlag der psychiatrischen Klinik; 1903.

[71] Foerster O. Zur pathogenese und chirurgischen Behandlung der Epilepsie. Zentralbl Chir 1925;52:531–49.

[72] Foerster O, Altenburger H. Electrobiologische Vorgänge an der menschlichen Hirnrinde. Dtsch Z Nervenheilkd 1935;135:277–88.

[73] Berger H. Über das Elektroenkephalogramm des Menschen. Arch Psychiatr Nervenkr 1929;87:527–70.

[74] Foerster O, Penfield W. The structural basis of traumatic epilepsy and results of radical operation. Brain 1930;53:99–119.

[75] Foerster O. The motor cortex in man in the light of Hughlings Jackson's doctrines. Brain 1936;59:135–59.

Chapter 2

Epidemiology of posttraumatic epilepsy

Overview

Posttraumatic epilepsy (PTE) refers to chronic unprovoked seizures following traumatic brain injury (TBI) and is a major clinical problem in both the military and civilian populations [1–3]. PTE is a common late complication of TBI. In this chapter, we review the epidemiology of PTE. First, we review the military studies of various forms of combat-associated head trauma and their association with the development of posttraumatic epilepsy that have been reported over the decades. Second, we review the analogous studies of posttraumatic epilepsy in civilian populations. Third, we evaluate risk factors based on the available studies. Fourth, we consider location of lesions. Fifth, we outline the natural history of PTE, including clinical heterogeneity, latency, and age-related factors.

Military injuries

Military conflicts have provided a rich source of data regarding the relationship between specific types of head injuries and the subsequent development of PTE. Overall, data from military conflicts indicate that PTE is reported in approximately one-third of war injuries with head trauma. This rate is remarkably similar when compared across 20th- and 21st-century wars (Table 2.1).

Nineteenth century war data

Very fragmentary data are available from 19th-century military conflicts [12]. Also, the accuracy of retrospective statistics from any past wars is open to criticism. Out of 167 Civil War (1861–65) skull wounds that were on the pension list, 14% had epilepsy, and out of 571 soldiers with gunshot wounds sustained in the Franco-Prussian War (1870–71), 4% developed epilepsy [13].

World War I data

Credner [4] studied 1990 German cases of war injuries with head trauma. Years examined were 1914–28. PTE was reported in 38%. In those with intact dura, the incidence was 19%; with dural penetration, the incidence was 49% [4].

Posttraumatic Epilepsy. https://doi.org/10.1016/B978-0-323-90099-7.00001-0

TABLE 2.1 Incidence of posttraumatic epilepsy (PTE) in combat injuries.

Study	Type of head injury (incidence)				Conflict	Follow-up (years)
	CHI	PHI	Total	Population (*n*)		
1. Credner [4]	19	50	38	1990	WWI	5
2. Walker and Jablon [5]	14	36	28	267	WWII	10
3. Caveness and Liss [6]	16	40	24	273	KW	5
4. Evans [7]	10–20	42	32	493	KW	11
5. Caveness [8]	20	50	31	273	KW	10
6. Salazar et al. [9]	–	53	–	421	VW	15
7. Eftekhar et al. [10]	–	74.7[a]	–	189	IR-IRW	21
8. Raymont et al. [11]	–	43.7	–	199	VW	35

[a] Percentage of persistent seizures (% of patients with seizures occurring in the past 2 years when observed 21 years after war trauma).
CHI, closed head injury. Mean value of incidence of seizures for CHI = 16.8%.
PHI, penetrating head injury. Mean value of incidence of seizures for PHI = 49.38%.
Overall mean value of incidence of seizures in any type of injuries (excluding studies 6 and 7) = 30.6%.
IR-IRW, Iraq-Iran War (1980–88); KW, Korean War; VW, Vietnam War; WWI, World War I; WWII, World War II.
Reproduced with permission from Da Silva AM, Willmore LJ. Posttraumatic epilepsy. In: Stefan H, Theodore WH, editors. Handbook of Clinical Neurology, Vol. 108 (3rd series) Epilepsy, Part II. Elsevier; 2012. p. 585–99.

On the British side, Ascroft studied 317 cases of gunshot wounds (GSW) to the head during World War I. With a 7–20-year follow-up, PTE was reported in 34%. In those with intact dura, the incidence was 23%; with dural penetration, the incidence was 45% [14].

World War II data

In 1947, A. Earl Walker (neurosurgeon at Johns Hopkins) and Seymour Jablon (statistician at the National Academy of Sciences-National Research Council), under the auspices of the Veterans Administration, decided to examine a series of 932 men who had sustained head injuries in World War II. Overall, 739 men were analyzed completely and the overall incidence of "convulsive episodes" was 28% [5]. Interestingly, this report detailed that there were many "types of attacks" ranging from generalized convulsions to focal manifestations associated with generalized seizures; but also there were cases of focal convulsions that never progressed to generalized convulsions. In terms of latency, approximately half of the patients who developed epilepsy had their first seizure within 9 months of injury. This study was notable in analyzing electroencephalography (EEG) in PTE for the first time, although no consistent EEG abnormalities were found in the PTE population studied [5]. In August 1961, Walker and Jablon published a full-length VA Medical Monograph entitled *A Follow-up Study of Head Wounds in World War II* in which they detailed many more clinical aspects of these cases including neurological deficits, types of seizures, electroencephalography, pneumoencephalography, and psychometry [15].

In 1951 and 1952, Russell and Whitty reported studies of World War II gunshot wounds with dural penetration seen at the Military Hospital in Oxford or at British mobile neurosurgical units. In this series of 830 men, in the first 5 years following injury PTE had developed in 43% [16,17]. The type of seizure was generalized in 53.9%, focal and generalized in 33.2%, and focal alone in 12.9% [16,17].

Korean War data

William Caveness and Henry Liss conducted a study of Korean War head injury casualties. In an initial study of 407 men (273 with closed head injury and 134 with penetrating head injury), they found an overall incidence of PTE of 23.8% (15.7% in the closed head injury group and 40.3% in the penetrating head injury group) [6]. In another study, Caveness studied 356 Korean War injuries, age 17–24, seen between 1951 and 1954 (8–11-year follow-up). 56% were missile injuries, and 44% were nonmissile head injuries. 109/356 (31%) developed PTE. In the subgroup of dura mater penetration with neurological deficit, the incidence of PTE was 55% (61/110) [8].

Evans reported on 422 veterans of the Korean War who sustained injuries. PTE followed in 32% of missile wounds and 8% of nonmissile wounds, and in 1 blast injury [7]. The incidence of PTE in the subset of missile wounds in which the brain was penetrated was 42% [7]. In this study, the incidence of

PTE was positively correlated with complications of the wound such as infection or hematoma, duration of unconsciousness or posttraumatic amnesia, and the presence of focal neurological signs. Evans provides some detailed clinical examples of PTE. In some cases, the focal seizures appeared to be precipitated by a voluntary movement of the part of the body in which the seizure began:

Example 1 A 21-year-old corporal sustained a left parietal penetrating wound from a grenade fragment. On regaining consciousness 5 h later he was dysphasic and had a right hemiplegia. Seven years later a mild right hemiparesis was the only residual sign. Focal motor seizures began 5 months after the injury, and they were frequently precipitated by reaching out his right arm for a newspaper or lifting a glass of water to his lips.

Example 2 A 23-year-old sailor shot himself in the left frontal region, causing prolonged stupor followed by confusion and emotional lability but no other neurological signs. Three years later he was at work and appeared well adjusted. Generalized seizures began 4 months after the injury, and more recently he had a number of focal seizures precipitated by turning his head too far to the right. "I could not turn my head back, and suddenly it began to twitch. I lost my power of speech but was aware of everything that went on around me." The attacks lasted for about 5 min.

In some cases, emotional stress appeared to trigger the posttraumatic seizures:

Example 3 A 21-year-old soldier fell 30 ft to the ground, sustaining a left parietal laceration but no fracture, and was unconscious for an hour. On the second day after the injury he noticed a twitching of his left lower eyelid which continued intermittently for a day or two. He then remained well until nearly 7 years later when, while waiting to appear in court to answer a criminal charge, he developed a "tic in my face which I couldn't control, then a jerking of the head." He then lost consciousness, falling to the ground in a major seizure. No other seizures have occurred.

In 1962, William Caveness, A. Earl Walker, and Peter Ascroft published a one-of-a-kind comparative study comparing the incidence of PTE in World War I, World War II, and the Korean War. This indicated a remarkably similar incidence: 32% following World War I, 34% following World War II, and 31% following the Korean War [18].

Vietnam War data

In 1979, Caveness and colleagues published a study of Vietnam War veterans. From a 1967–70 roster of 1250 head-injured Vietnam War veterans, which included a registry of type and extent of head injury, they analyzed 1030 cases from July 1976 to July 1978. PTE incidence in this group was 344/1030 (33%) [2]. In addition, they analyzed latency to seizure onset in this group and found 40%–50% occurred by 6 months, 70% by 1 year, and 80% of cases by 2 years [2]. In a follow-up report, they devised a mathematical formula to describe the onset of first seizures after injury to help practitioners assess prognostic indicators [19].

In 1985, Salazar and colleagues published a report from the Vietnam Head Injury Study (VHIS). The VHIS is a prospective, longitudinal follow-up of Vietnam War veterans with mostly penetrating head injuries. An early report of 421 veterans who had penetrating brain wounds in Vietnam ~ 15 years prior demonstrated that 53% had posttraumatic epilepsy, and one-half of those still had seizures 15 years after injury [9]. These investigators conveyed the message that earlier investigations of PTE did not include a long enough follow-up period to detect the very late-onset seizures [20]. A long-term follow-up study of patients from the Vietnam Head Injury Study was published in 2010 [11]. This report had a number of interesting findings, including: (1) the prevalence of seizures (43.7%) was similar to that found during phase 2 evaluations 20 years earlier, but 11 of 87 (12.6%) reported very late onset of PTE after phase 2 (more than 14 years after injury); (2) within the phase 3 cohort, the most common seizure type last experienced was complex partial seizures (31.0%), with increasing frequency after injury; (3) of subjects with PTE, 88% were receiving anticonvulsants; (4) left parietal lobe lesions and retained ferric metal fragments were associated with PTE in a logistic regression model; and (5) total brain volume loss predicted seizure frequency. The authors conclude that patients with penetrating head injury carry risk for PTE development even decades after TBI [11].

Overall, in spite of other changes in medical care from 1914 to 1970, a similar incidence of PTE has been observed across all 20th-century wars [2].

Other more recent war data

In 2009, Eftekhar *et al.* from the Sina Trauma Research Center in Tehran, Iran, reported a retrospective study of 189 Iranian casualties from the Iraq-Iran War (1980–88) [10]. They explicitly selected a subgroup of Iraq-Iran War veterans who had sustained penetrating head injury and had already exhibited PTE. The probability of persistent seizures in different periods after injury was estimated using Kaplan-Meier analysis. The mean time since injury in this patient population was 18.6 ± 4.7 years. Probability of persistent seizures was 86.4% after 16 years and 74.7% after 21 years [10]. The authors found that early seizures, prophylactic antiepileptic drugs, and surgical intervention did not significantly affect long-term outcome in terms of seizure persistence. This study highlights the long-term persistence of PTE in military populations with penetrating head injury once it develops.

In 2014, Chen *et al.* reported on PTE incidence in a cohort of 16 US veterans from Operation Enduring Freedom (OEF) and Operation Iraqi Freedom (OIF) [21]. This study was carried out at the VA Greater Los Angeles Healthcare System. Inclusion criteria were all OEF/OIF veterans who had both TBI and seizures diagnosed between October 1, 2007, and September 30, 2009. Seizures were determined from VA medical records and encompassed both epileptic seizures and psychogenic nonepileptic seizures (PNES). All veterans were male with a mean age of 30 years. Of importance, in these wars, blast exposure was the most common mechanism of TBI (81%). This distinguishes some recent wars from 20th-century wars (above). Although all veterans were assigned a diagnosis code of seizures, the diagnosis of PTE was clinically confirmed in only 3 veterans, whereas the diagnosis of posttraumatic stress disorder was confirmed in 81% and a diagnosis of PNES was suspected in 44% [21]. While not conclusive based on a small sample, this study suggests that blast TBI may not lead to epileptic seizures nearly as frequently as impact-based closed head injury or penetrating head injury. This is borne out in animal studies in which blast injury is not associated with PTE to the same extent as other models of injury such as controlled cortical impact (CCI) (Chapters 6 and 7).

In 2015, Pugh *et al.* reported a cross-sectional observational study of Afghanistan (OEF) and Iraq (OIF) veterans who received inpatient and outpatient care in the Veterans Health Administration in the year 2009–10 [22]. Of 256,284 veterans, 2719 (or 10.6 per 1000) were found to have epilepsy. A statistically significant association was found between epilepsy and prior TBI diagnosis. The strongest association was in the subgroup with penetrating TBI [22].

Civilian injuries

In the civilian population, the incidence of PTE is dependent on the severity of brain injury, and studies in distinct populations have reported a PTE incidence of 7%–32% [1,23–37] (Table 2.2). However, many of the studies report populations of civilian patients after severe TBI, and therein lies the heterogeneity in these studies. Also, of course, the causes of TBI in a civilian population are more heterogeneous, including falls, assaults, and motor vehicle accidents [39].

Influential population-based studies of PTE incidence after TBI were performed by Annegers and colleagues [1,26]. An early study involved 2747 head injury patients from Olmsted County, Minnesota, during the interval 1935 through 1974 who were followed to determine the risk of PTE [26]. Injuries were classified as severe (brain contusion, intracerebral or intracranial hematoma, or >24 h of unconsciousness or amnesia), moderate (skull fracture or 30 min to 24 h of unconsciousness or amnesia), and mild (briefer unconsciousness or amnesia). A subsequent study extended follow-up of this cohort and included additional cases from the period from 1975 through 1984 [1]. This latter study of 4541 children and adults with TBI occurring between 1935 and 1984 is the largest of its kind in the civilian population. The PTE incidence was 1.5% for mild TBI, 2.9% for moderate TBI, and 17% for severe TBI (Fig. 2.1). In the multivariate analysis, significant risk factors for PTE were brain contusion with subdural hematoma, skull fracture, loss of consciousness or amnesia for >24 h, and age 65 years or older [1]. Similar findings were obtained in a distinct population-based US study following 2118 patients hospitalized with TBI [40].

In aggregate, the studies reveal that the severe TBI civilian population (Table 2.2) approaches but does not reach the PTE incidence in military TBI

TABLE 2.2 Incidence of posttraumatic epilepsy (PTE) in civilian injuries.

Study	Incidence of PTE (%)	Population (n)	Follow-up (years)
Studies in general (mainly adult) population			
1. Jennett [24]	7.5	240[a]	4 (early seizures excluded)
2. Caveness [25]	14–15	1.9 million[a]	3 (severe trauma[a])
3. Annegers et al. [26]	11.6	2747	5
4. Guidice and Berchou [27]	25	164[a]	1 (severe trauma[a])
5. Ogunniyi et al. [28]	9	1551[a]	15 months
6. Al-Rajeh et al. [29]	11	1000[a]	4
7. Martins da Silva et al. [30]	10	506	5
8. Burcet and Olabe [38]	7	23082[a]	10
9. Asikainen et al. [31]	25.3	490	5 to >20
10. Englander et al. [32]	10	647	up to 2 (167 less than 2 years old)
11. Skandsen et al. [33]	23	93	3–8
Studies in children			
12. Black et al. [34]	10	307	6
13. Foulon and Noel [35]	11	244[a]	5 (early seizures[a])
14. Annegers et al. [26][b]	30	2747	5
15. Lundar and Nestvold [36]	7	126	5
16. Kieslich and Jacobi [37]	20.6	318	2–8
17. Asikainen et al. [31][c]	31.9	490	5 to >20
18. Skandsen et al. [33][d]	16	91	3–8

[a]Population-based study not specifically evaluating head trauma. Overall mean value of incidence of PTE = 13.99%.
[b]Children cohort analysis based on data from study 3. Overall mean value of incidence of PTE = 15.81%.
[c]This study (also reported in study 9) includes a cohort of 241 children (up to 16 years old). 77 of whom had "late PTE."
[d]This study (also reported in study 11) includes data from children aged up to 19 years that are not matched in other series.
Reproduced with permission from Da Silva AM, Willmore LJ. Posttraumatic epilepsy. In: Stefan H, Theodore WH, editors. Handbook of Clinical Neurology, Vol. 108 (3rd series) Epilepsy, Part II. Elsevier; 2012. p. 585–99.

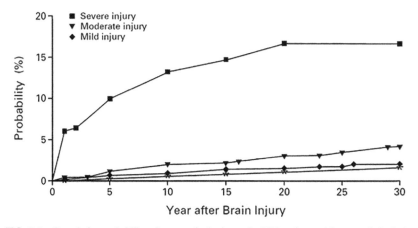

FIG. 2.1 Cumulative probability of unprovoked seizures in 4541 patients with traumatic brain injuries, according to the severity of the injury and the incidence of seizures in the general population. *(Reproduced with permission from Annegers JF, et al. A population-based study of seizures after traumatic brain injuries. N Engl J Med 1998;338(1):20–24.)*

studies of PTE (Table 2.1). W.B. Jennett conducted a series of studies of PTE in civilians admitted with head injuries to the Radcliffe Infirmary, Oxford [24,41–43]. In 1000 patients studied, a subset was followed for at least 4 years with various types of injury. Incidence of late seizures (PTE) was associated with presence of early posttraumatic seizures (within the first week after injury), prolonged posttraumatic amnesia (>24 h duration), and severity of injury (in particular presence of depressed skull fracture or intracranial hematoma) [24,41–43].

Risk factors

Risk factors for PTE (summarizing military and civilian studies) include severity of trauma, penetrating head injuries, intracranial hematoma, depressed skull fracture, prolonged unconsciousness (>24 h), and early posttraumatic seizures [31,44–46] (Table 2.3). In the subset with penetrating head injuries,

---

TABLE 2.3 Risk factors for development of posttraumatic epilepsy.

Severity of trauma
Penetrating head injury
Intracranial hematoma
Depressed skull fracture
Prolonged unconsciousness (>24 h)
Early posttraumatic seizures

PTE risk nears 50% in most studies (Table 2.1). Individual studies also have identified other distinct risk factors in specific cohorts studied. For example, in the VHIS PTE predictive factors included cortical involvement, a moderate volume of brain tissue loss, intracerebral hematoma, and retained metal fragments [9]. Other studies also indicated that prolonged posttraumatic amnesia, presence of cortical laceration associated with a depressed skull fracture, and intracerebral hematoma are independent risk factors [41,47]. Civilian studies most clearly indicated that severity of injury was the most important single risk factor [1,26].

In 2003, Englander et al. reported the risk of PTE in a cohort of patients evaluated in a prospective, observational study of patients with moderate to severe TBI admitted to 4 trauma centers within 24 h of injury [32]. A total of 647 individuals (16 years of age or older) were enrolled from August 1993 through September 1997 and followed for up to 24 months. Of this group, 66 individuals had late posttraumatic seizures. Interestingly, the highest cumulative probability for late posttraumatic seizures included biparietal contusions, dural penetration with bone and metal fragments, multiple intracranial operations, multiple subcortical contusions, subdural hematoma with evacuation, midline shift >5 mm, and multiple cortical contusions. This study provided more granular detail on individual anatomic and imaging risk factors for PTE in specific TBI subgroups [32]. The authors' main overall conclusion was "the amount of focal tissue destruction is the most important factor in predicting the development of late posttraumatic seizure" [32].

Sports-related concussions and posttraumatic epilepsy

An estimated 283,000 children seek care in US emergency departments each year for a sports- or recreation-related TBI [48]. TBIs sustained in contact sports account for ~45% of these visits. Football, bicycling, basketball, playground activities, and soccer account for the highest number of emergency department visits [48]. Thus, sports-related concussions (SRCs) may represent a specific type of TBI to be evaluated as a risk factor for PTE, as convulsions occur in an estimated 1 in 70 concussions [49]. While little study has been given to SRCs as a risk factor for PTE, illustrative cases have been reported. In 2020, Hellwinkel et al. reported the case of a 15-year-old male football player who sustained multiple SRCs [50]. He had a witnessed tonic-clonic seizure, subsequent postconcussive symptomatology, and several more tonic-clonic seizures in the several months postinjury, thus satisfying the criteria for PTE [50]. A recent comprehensive review reported on 130 athletes with SRC-associated convulsions; over an average follow-up period of 3.3 years, 9 (6.9%) developed new-onset epilepsy (i.e. PTE) [49]. Overall, the prevalence of PTE in athletes is probably underestimated due to the underreporting of concussive symptoms [51]. Clearly, large-scale studies are needed to more fully examine SRCs as a risk factor for PTE.

Natural history

Location of lesions

Of course, the mechanism and severity of TBI in any individual case will determine the location, extent, and multiplicity of brain lesions potentially responsible for PTE. Combat injuries tend to predominate over the central external convexity with motor or sensory cortex involved [52]. Interestingly, some earlier military studies suggested that parietal lesion location conferred more susceptibility to PTE [6,17]. However, civilian TBI more commonly involves contusions in the frontal and temporal lobes [45,53–55]. In the temporal lobe, seizures may arise from the neocortex or mesial temporal structures. Hemorrhagic temporal lobe injuries are associated with a particularly high rate of PTE development [45]. In a study of 23 patients with PTE, 11 (48%) had seizures arising from the neocortex and 8 (35%) had mesial temporal sclerosis on magnetic resonance imaging [56]. In cortical contusions (intraparenchymal hematomas), blood products (*e.g.* hemosiderin) can accumulate and lead to focal epileptogenic cysts [57,58]. In the case of penetrating injury, seizures tend to originate from adjacent injured cortex [30].

Clinical heterogeneity

Heterogeneity of injury severity and location is paralleled by clinical heterogeneity of PTE manifestation [59]. The issue of whether early posttraumatic seizures predict late seizures (*i.e.* PTE) has been extensively studied, but results are conflicting [60]. Risk factors for early and late seizures are similar, and a large population-based study found that early seizures are not an independent risk factor for late seizures (PTE) [1]. What is clear, however, based on many studies is that the development of PTE after TBI may have a long latency. In general, >80% of PTE begins within 2 years of TBI but the relative risk for developing PTE remains elevated long after the inciting injury in both adults [11] and children [61,62]. This prolonged period of posttraumatic epileptogenesis presents the opportunity for antiepileptic prophylaxis (Chapter 4).

Another aspect of PTE heterogeneity concerns seizure subtypes. It has been thought that early seizures after TBI are mostly generalized tonic-clonic [63], whereas late seizures are more likely to be focal in onset [55]. However, continuous EEG monitoring in the intensive care unit (ICU) has revealed many nonconvulsive seizures early after TBI [64]. These findings suggest that "the more you look the more you find" in terms of epileptiform abnormalities and nonconvulsive seizures early after TBI [65]. Regarding the late seizures (*i.e.* PTE), most PTE patients have seizures that are focal with secondary generalization [32,55], but predominantly focal seizures may also occur [56,59]. Animal models of PTE tend to recapitulate the focal seizures without generalization (Chapters 6 and 7).

A final aspect of PTE heterogeneity is that the incidence and prevalence of PTE differ among age groups [23]. In general, the range of incidence of

PTE in children is greater than in adults (7%–30%) (Table 2.2) [34]. Children younger than 2 years appear to have the greatest incidence [66]. A retrospective study of children with severe TBI concluded that in addition to injury severity as defined by the Glasgow Coma Scale (GCS) score, type of trauma and brain lesion, hypoxia, hypotension, hyperglycemia, and early posttraumatic seizures influence outcome [67]. In one series of 318 children with head injury of sufficient severity to require hospitalization, 19.8% had early seizures and 21.4% developed PTE [37]. The overall incidence appears to be lower in long-term follow-up studies of pediatric patients with mild TBI (mTBI). In one study of children 0–17 years of age admitted to a single medical center between 2007 and 2009 with a diagnosis of mTBI, the overall incidence of PTE was 3.1% [62]. Interestingly, the mean time between trauma and onset of seizures was 3.1 years in this study, indicating a longer latency in this pediatric population than in most adult studies. Other pediatric studies have also suggested a longer latency between brain injury and first late seizure [31], suggesting the need for longitudinal studies of greater duration in the pediatric population.

In contrast to the pediatric population, PTE in the elderly has been poorly studied. However, the incidence of seizures and epilepsy is highest in subjects older than 65 due to epileptogenic brain insults and diseases [68]. Head trauma accounts for up to 20% of epilepsy in the elderly, and age of 65 years or more has been identified as one of the risk factors for developing epilepsy after a head injury [69–71]. Older individuals are at increased risk of head injuries and resultant TBI due to falls. Intracranial hemorrhage (including subdural and intraparenchymal hemorrhage) is a strong risk factor for PTE in the aging population. In addition, TBI in the elderly may be superimposed upon age-related alterations in the function of the neurovascular unit (NVU) [72].

References

[1] Annegers JF, et al. A population-based study of seizures after traumatic brain injuries. N Engl J Med 1998;338(1):20–4.

[2] Caveness WF, et al. The nature of posttraumatic epilepsy. J Neurosurg 1979;50(5):545–53.

[3] Lowenstein DH. Epilepsy after head injury: an overview. Epilepsia 2009;50(Suppl 2):4–9.

[4] Credner L. Klinische und soziale Auswirkungen von Hirnschädigungen. Z Ges Neurol Psychiatr 1930;126:721–57.

[5] Walker AE, Jablon S. A follow-up of head injured men of World War II. J Neurosurg 1959;16:600–10.

[6] Caveness WF, Liss HR. Incidence of post-traumatic epilepsy. Epilepsia 1961;2:123–9.

[7] Evans JH. Posttraumatic epilepsy. Neurology 1962;12:665–74.

[8] Caveness WF. Onset and cessation of fits following craniocerebral trauma. J Neurosurg 1963;20:570–83.

[9] Salazar AM, et al. Epilepsy after penetrating head injury. I. Clinical correlates: a report of the Vietnam head injury study. Neurology 1985;35(10):1406–14.

[10] Eftekhar B, et al. Prognostic factors in the persistence of posttraumatic epilepsy after penetrating head injuries sustained in war. J Neurosurg 2009;110(2):319–26.

[11] Raymont V, et al. Correlates of posttraumatic epilepsy 35 years following combat brain injury. Neurology 2010;75(3):224–9.

[12] Friedlander WJ. The history of modern epilepsy: the beginning, 1865–1914. Westport, CT: Greenwood Press; 2001.

[13] Allen D, Sanford H, Dolley D. Traumatic defects of the skull. Their relation to epilepsy. A clinical and experimental study of their repair. Boston Med Surg J 1906;154:396–405.

[14] Ascroft PB. Traumatic epilepsy after gunshot wounds of the head. Br Med J 1941;1:739–44.

[15] Walker AE, Jablon S. Follow-up study of head wounds in World War II., 1961, Washington, DC: The National Academies Press.

[16] Russell WR. Disability caused by brain wounds. J Neurol Neurosurg Psychiatry 1951;14:35–9.

[17] Russell WR, Whitty CWM. Studies in traumatic epilepsy. Part 1 (Factors influencing the incidence of epilepsy after brain wounds). J Neurol Neurosurg Psychiatry 1952;15:93–8.

[18] Caveness WF, Walker AE, Ascroft PB. Incidence of posttraumatic epilepsy in Korean veterans as compared with those from World War I and World War II. J Neurosurg 1962;19:122–9.

[19] Weiss GH, et al. Prognostic factors for the occurrence of posttraumatic epilepsy. Arch Neurol 1983;40(1):7–10.

[20] Weiss GH, et al. Predicting posttraumatic epilepsy in penetrating head injury. Arch Neurol 1986;43(8):771–3.

[21] Chen LL, et al. Posttraumatic epilepsy in operation enduring freedom/operation Iraqi freedom veterans. Mil Med 2014;179(5):492–6.

[22] Pugh MJ, et al. The prevalence of epilepsy and association with traumatic brain injury in veterans of the Afghanistan and Iraq wars. J Head Trauma Rehabil 2015;30(1):29–37.

[23] Da Silva AM, Willmore LJ. Posttraumatic epilepsy. In: Stefan H, Theodore WH, editors. Handbook of clinical neurology, vol. 108 (3rd series) Epilepsy, Part II. Elsevier; 2012. p. 585–99.

[24] Jennett WB. Early traumatic epilepsy. Definition and identity. Lancet 1969;1(7604):1023–5.

[25] Caveness WF. Epilepsy, a product of trauma in our time. Epilepsia 1976;17(2):207–15.

[26] Annegers JF, et al. Seizures after head trauma: a population study. Neurology 1980;30(7 Pt 1):683–9.

[27] Guidice MA, Berchou RC. Post-traumatic epilepsy following head injury. Brain Inj 1987;1(1):61–4.

[28] Ogunniyi A, et al. Risk factors for epilepsy: case-control study in Nigerians. Epilepsia 1987;28(3):280–5.

[29] Al-Rajeh S, et al. Epilepsy and other convulsive disorders in Saudi Arabia: a prospective study of 1,000 consecutive cases. Acta Neurol Scand 1990;82(5):341–5.

[30] da Silva AM, et al. Controversies in posttraumatic epilepsy. Acta Neurochir Suppl (Wien) 1990;50:48–51.

[31] Asikainen I, Kaste M, Sarna S. Early and late posttraumatic seizures in traumatic brain injury rehabilitation patients: brain injury factors causing late seizures and influence of seizures on long-term outcome. Epilepsia 1999;40(5):584–9.

[32] Englander J, et al. Analyzing risk factors for late posttraumatic seizures: a prospective, multi-center investigation. Arch Phys Med Rehabil 2003;84(3):365–73.

[33] Skandsen T, et al. Global outcome, productivity and epilepsy 3-8 years after severe head injury. The impact of injury severity. Clin Rehabil 2008;22(7):653–62.

[34] Black P, Shepard R, Walker AE. Outcome of head trauma: age and posttraumatic seizures. In: Porter R, Fitzsimon DW, editors. Outcome of severe damage to the central nervous system. Amsterdam: Elsevier; 1975. p. 215–26.

[35] Foulon M, Noel P. Epilepsie post-traumatique precoce dans l'enfance: signification et prognostic a court terme. Acta Neurol Belg 1977;77:276–84.

[36] Lundar T, Nestvold K. Pediatric head injuries caused by traffic accidents. A prospective study with 5-year follow-up. Childs Nerv Syst 1985;1(1):24–8.

[37] Kieslich M, Jacobi G. Incidence and risk factors of post-traumatic epilepsy in childhood. Lancet 1995;345(8943):187.

[38] Burcet-Darde J, Olabe Jauregui J. Estudio epidemiologico de la epilepsia posttraumatica en la isla de Mallorca. Neurologia (Spain) 1992;7:49–51.

[39] Christensen J. The epidemiology of posttraumatic epilepsy. Semin Neurol 2015;35(3):218–22.

[40] Ferguson PL, et al. A population-based study of risk of epilepsy after hospitalization for traumatic brain injury. Epilepsia 2010;51(5):891–8.

[41] Jennett WB. Late epilepsy after blunt head injuries: a clinical study based on 282 cases of traumatic epilepsy. Ann R Coll Surg Engl 1961;29:370–84.

[42] Jennett WB, Lewin W. Traumatic epilepsy after closed head injuries. J Neurol Neurosurg Psychiatry 1960;23:295–301.

[43] Jennett WB. Predicting epilepsy after blunt head injury. Br Med J 1965;1(5444):1215–6.

[44] Garga N, Lowenstein DH. Posttraumatic epilepsy: a major problem in desperate need of major advances. Epilepsy Curr 2006;6(1):1–5.

[45] Tubi MA, et al. Early seizures and temporal lobe trauma predict post-traumatic epilepsy: a longitudinal study. Neurobiol Dis 2019;123:115–21.

[46] Temkin NR. Risk factors for posttraumatic seizures in adults. Epilepsia 2003;44(s10):18–20.

[47] Jennett B. Epilepsy and acute traumatic intracranial haematoma. J Neurol Neurosurg Psychiatry 1975;38(4):378–81.

[48] Sarmiento K, et al. Emergency department visits for sports- and recreation-related traumatic brain injuries among children—United States, 2010-2016. MMWR Morb Mortal Wkly Rep 2019;68(10):237–42.

[49] Kuhl NO, et al. Sport-related concussive convulsions: a systematic review. Phys Sportsmed 2018;46(1):1–7.

[50] Hellwinkel JE, et al. Post-traumatic epilepsy after sports-related concussion: a case report. Neurotrauma Rep 2020;1(1):42–5.

[51] Wallace J, et al. Knowledge of concussion and reporting behaviors in high school athletes with or without access to an athletic trainer. J Athl Train 2017;52(3):228–35.

[52] Feeney DM, Walker AE. The prediction of posttraumatic epilepsy. A mathematical approach. Arch Neurol 1979;36(1):8–12.

[53] Payan H, Toga M, Berard-Badier M. The pathology of post-traumatic epilepsies. Epilepsia 1970;11(1):81–94.

[54] Marks DA, et al. Seizure localization and pathology following head injury in patients with uncontrolled epilepsy. Neurology 1995;45(11):2051–7.

[55] Gupta PK, et al. Subtypes of post-traumatic epilepsy: clinical, electrophysiological, and imaging features. J Neurotrauma 2014;31(16):1439–43.

[56] Diaz-Arrastia R, et al. Neurophysiologic and neuroradiologic features of intractable epilepsy after traumatic brain injury in adults. Arch Neurol 2000;57(11):1611–6.

[57] Willmore LJ, Sypert GW, Munson JB. Recurrent seizures induced by cortical iron injection: a model of posttraumatic epilepsy. Ann Neurol 1978;4(4):329–36.

[58] Willmore LJ, et al. Chronic focal epileptiform discharges induced by injection of iron into rat and cat cortex. Science 1978;200(4349):1501–3.

[59] Diaz-Arrastia R, et al. Posttraumatic epilepsy: the endophenotypes of a human model of epileptogenesis. Epilepsia 2009;50(Suppl 2):14–20.

[60] Rao VR, Parko KL. Clinical approach to posttraumatic epilepsy. Semin Neurol 2015;35(1):57–63.

[61] Hung R, et al. Systematic review of the clinical course, natural history, and prognosis for pediatric mild traumatic brain injury: results of the International Collaboration on Mild Traumatic Brain Injury Prognosis. Arch Phys Med Rehabil 2014;95(3 Suppl):S174–91.

[62] Keret A, et al. Posttraumatic epilepsy: long-term follow-up of children with mild traumatic brain injury. J Neurosurg Pediatr 2017;20(1):64–70.

[63] Lee ST, Lui TN. Early seizures after mild closed head injury. J Neurosurg 1992;76(3):435–9.

[64] Vespa PM, et al. Increased incidence and impact of nonconvulsive and convulsive seizures after traumatic brain injury as detected by continuous electroencephalographic monitoring. J Neurosurg 1999;91(5):750–60.

[65] Nuwer MR, et al. Routine and quantitative EEG in mild traumatic brain injury. Clin Neurophysiol 2005;116(9):2001–25.

[66] Kieslich M, et al. Neurological and mental outcome after severe head injury in childhood: a long-term follow-up of 318 children. Disabil Rehabil 2001;23(15):665–9.

[67] Chiaretti A, et al. Prognostic factors and outcome of children with severe head injury: an 8-year experience. Childs Nerv Syst 2002;18(3–4):129–36.

[68] Sen A, et al. Epilepsy in older people. Lancet 2020;395(10225):735–48.

[69] Acharya JN, Acharya VJ. Epilepsy in the elderly: special considerations and challenges. Ann Indian Acad Neurol 2014;17(Suppl 1):S18–26.

[70] Brodie MJ, Elder AT, Kwan P. Epilepsy in later life. Lancet Neurol 2009;8(11):1019–30.

[71] Stefan H. Epilepsy in the elderly: facts and challenges. Acta Neurol Scand 2011;124(4):223–37.

[72] van Vliet EA, Marchi N. Neurovascular unit dysfunction as a mechanism of seizures and epilepsy during aging. Epilepsia 2022;63:1297–1313.

Chapter 3

Neuropathology of posttraumatic epilepsy

Overview

In this chapter, we review the neuropathology of posttraumatic epilepsy (PTE). First, we review the aspects of the career of Wilder Penfield. Penfield embodied the link from early neurosurgery through neurocytology to neuropathology and rational epilepsy surgery. Together with Otfrid Foerster, he was the first to carefully study pathological specimens from patients with posttraumatic epilepsy with the most modern histological techniques available at the time. Finally, we consider some more modern neuropathological issues related to traumatic brain injury (TBI) and PTE.

Wilder Penfield

To the modern neuroscientist, Wilder Penfield (1891–1976) (Fig. 3.1) needs a little introduction. Many are familiar with the basic outline of his legendary career (Table 3.1). Penfield is justifiably famous for two main achievements: his tremendous contributions to the functional mapping of the human brain in the surgical treatment of epilepsy and the founding of the Montreal Neurological Institute. However, lesser known but seminal as well was his initial neuropathological work examining and characterizing glial cells. The modern reader may be surprised that Penfield was, together with his Spanish mentor Pío Del Río-Hortega, the first to properly describe oligodendroglial cells [1,2].

In 1923, a young Wilder Penfield was attempting to stain brain scars in the laboratories of the New York-Presbyterian Hospital in the hope of identifying the mysterious cause of posttraumatic epilepsy in both animal models and humans. Penfield had begun this project 2 years earlier, when he began teaching medical students at the Columbia College of Physicians and Surgeons under the authority of William C. Clarke, professor of surgical pathology. Clarke challenged Penfield immediately, asking "Wouldn't you like to see how the nerve cells, and all the other cells that surround them and nourish them, behave when…you make an incision in the brain? What is the cause of epilepsy?" [3].

Penfield was fascinated by epilepsy from his very first exposure to the central nervous system (CNS), mentioning that as early as his undergraduate years, he "had filled [his] index cards with notes from the writings of Hughlings Jackson"

Posttraumatic Epilepsy. https://doi.org/10.1016/B978-0-323-90099-7.00002-2

43

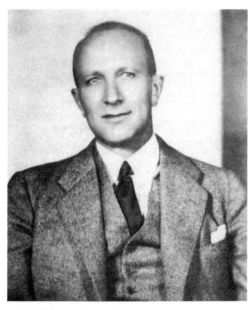

FIG. 3.1   Wilder Penfield (1891–1976). American neurosurgeon and neuroscientist. Made seminal contributions to neurohistology (codiscovering oligodendroglia with Río-Hortega). Studied wound healing in the brain and developed a neuropathological theory for the etiology of posttraumatic epilepsy. Pioneered awake brain mapping and epilepsy surgery. Founded the Montreal Neurological Institute. *(Reproduced with permission from Preul MC, Feindel W, Origins of Wilder Penfield's surgical technique: the role of the "Cushing ritual" and influences from the European experience. J Neurosurg 1991;75:812–820.)*

[3]. Clarke gave Penfield his first opportunity to begin studying the disease. He recognized immediately, however, "that the methods we use show only half the picture" [3], and indeed 2 years later, Penfield met a "dead end" in his work due to the inability to stain the nonneuronal cells of the CNS. Penfield believed these cells were crucial to demonstrating the healing process of the brain and in helping elucidate why a "healing scar so often leads to epilepsy" [3].

It was then that Penfield recalled the trouble he had staining neurons in the lab of another famous mentor he had worked with while on a Rhodes Scholarship, Sir Charles S. Sherrington of Oxford University (1857–1952) (Fig. 3.2), who had admonished him "Don't give up until you have tried the methods of Ramón y Cajal" [3]. (Sherrington had invited Cajal to stay at his home during Cajal's Croonian Lectureship in 1894 and the awarding of an honorary degree from Oxford; Cajal was rumored to have turned the guest bedroom into a histology laboratory! [4]). Remembering the brilliant success he had met with using Cajal's staining techniques, Penfield immediately went to the New York Academy of Medicine to read Cajal's articles in the hopes of adopting his staining techniques once again, only this time for glia rather than neurons. Although the techniques proved fruitful, Penfield was not able at first to emulate

TABLE 3.1 Some significant events in the life of Wilder Penfield.

Year(s)	Event
1904	At 13, Penfield discovers the existence of Rhodes Scholarship
1913	Graduation from Princeton
1914	Awarded Rhodes Scholarship
1915–16	Medical student at Oxford, exposed to William Osler and Charles Sherrington
1916–18	Johns Hopkins Medical School
1918–19	Surgical internship at Peter Bent Brigham Hospital, Boston
1919–20	Returned to Oxford for postgraduate study. Works with Sherrington assistants Cuthbert Bazett on decerebrate rigidity, and Harry M. Carleton on neurocytology
1921	Joins staff as a neurosurgeon at Presbyterian Hospital, New York (surgical chief: Allen Whipple)
1924	Leaves Presbyterian Hospital to go to Madrid
September 1924	Returns to New York and Presbyterian Hospital, meets William Vernon Cone and inaugurates Laboratory of Neurocytology
1928	Works with Otfrid Foerster in Breslau, Germany for 6 months
1928	Arrives in Montreal (Royal Victoria Hospital and McGill University)
December 11, 1928	Operates on sister Ruth for oligodendroglioma
1932	Publishes *Cytology and Cellular Pathology of the Nervous System*, a 3-volume text with contributions from world-leading authorities, many of whom Penfield knew personally
September 27, 1934	Opening of the Montreal Neurological Institute

the beautiful stains of Cajal's greatest disciple, Pío Del Río-Hortega, nor was he able to completely interpret the results of the stains he used.

In January of 1924, Penfield decided to approach the man who had recruited him to the Presbyterian Hospital, surgical chief and professor of surgery Allen O. Whipple (Fig. 3.3), in the hopes of securing funds to travel to Spain and study under Pío Del Río-Hortega. Río-Hortega had published detailed drawings

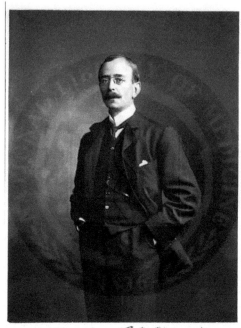

C. S. Sherrington

FIG. 3.2 Charles S. Sherrington (1857–1952). English neurophysiologist, histologist, bacteriologist, and pathologist. Introduced the term "synapse" and explained synaptic communication between neurons. Described the nature and functions of reflexes. Published *The Integrative Action of the Nervous System* in 1906. Received the Nobel Prize in Physiology or Medicine in 1932 with Edgar Adrian for their work on the functions of neurons. *(Reproduced with permission from Gill AS, Binder DK. Wilder Penfield, Pío del Río-Hortega, and the discovery of oligodendroglia, Neurosurgery 2007;60(5):940–48.)*

of the nonneuronal cells that Penfield stated were "no more than ghosts" [3] in his preparations. Although Penfield was unsure how Whipple would respond, Whipple was quite supportive and decided to call upon Mrs. Percy Rockefeller. He had operated on her daughter free of charge and was able to secure a generous grant from Mrs. Rockefeller. With the help of a few other benefactors, Whipple secured enough funds to allow for Penfield, his wife, and two children to spend 6 months in Madrid. Here, Penfield hoped to work closely with Río-Hortega to "study the brain of man, and then move on to the effects of disease on the brain" [3]. Interestingly, Penfield and family set sail for Spain before receiving any word or invitation from Río-Hortega. Penfield wryly describes finally receiving Río-Hortega's one-word imperative, "*venga*" ("come"), while halfway across the Atlantic [3].

It was not until the publication of the *reazione nera* ("black reaction" or silver stain) by Camillo Golgi (1843–1926) [8,9] that a means for the more exact study of nerve cells and neuroglia was made possible. Santiago Ramón y Cajal's pioneering

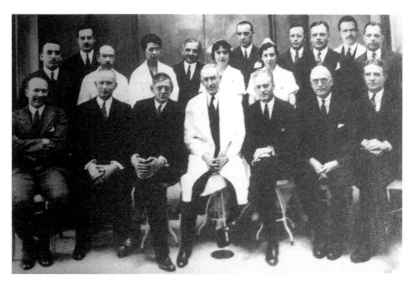

FIG. 3.3   Allen O. Whipple (center) and his surgical team, including Wilder Penfield (far left), c.1924 at the Presbyterian Hospital. William V. Cone is standing behind Penfield. Whipple was known for developing the pancreaticoduodenectomy ("Whipple procedure") and describing Whipple's triad (diagnostic triad for insulinoma). *(Reproduced with permission from Gill AS, Binder DK. Wilder Penfield, Pío del Río-Hortega, and the discovery of oligodendroglia, Neurosurgery 2007;60(5):940–48.)*

modifications of Golgi's technique made possible the detailed anatomical study of the central nervous system. In fact, Cajal's modifications and studies were so fundamental that many, including Sherrington and Penfield, regarded Cajal (Fig. 3.4) as the true father of neuroanatomy [3]. His studies on glial cells came after his celebrated studies of neurons. Using his new gold chloride-sublimate method, Cajal demonstrated the morphology of the protoplasmic neuroglia as well as the fibrous neuroglia of the white matter in 1913 [10,11]. Cajal also recognized that the "satellites" and "interfascicular cells" were of a different class from neuroglia, which he termed "*the third element*" [10].

However, the remainder of the "adventitial" or nonnervous cells remained unstained until Cajal's disciple Pío Del Río-Hortega (1882–1945) (Fig. 3.5) described a method of using silver carbonate to stain neuroglia and connective tissue in 1918 [12,13]. For the first time, this distinguished two cell types with distinct cytoplasmic expansions, which Río-Hortega termed microglia and oligodendroglia. Thus the nonneural interstitial cells could be divided into four classes: (1) fibrous neuroglia; (2) protoplasmic neuroglia; (3) microglia; and (4) oligodendroglia. Oligodendroglia were so named because they exhibited fewer (Greek *oligo*— few) and smaller branches (Greek *dendro*—branch) than astrocytes and were later called *oligodendrocytes* (as astroglia are *astrocytes*). Río-Hortega would go on to focus his research efforts on microglia, elucidating their genesis, function, and pathologies in a remarkably precise fashion [14]. He indicated that microglia are

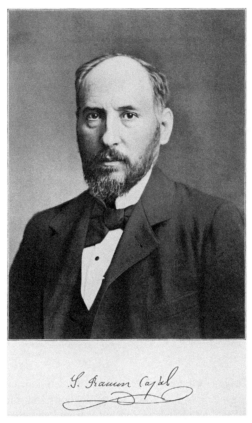

FIG. 3.4 Santiago Ramón y Cajal (1852–1934). Great Spanish neurohistologist. Worked in Valencia, Barcelona, and Madrid. Applied Golgi's method to study and describe in detail almost every part of the central nervous system. Cajal's studies provided overwhelming evidence in favor of the "neuron doctrine," which contrasted with the reticular theory [5,6]. Devoted his later career to investigation of pathological processes within the nervous system, summarized in a classic of neuroscience *Degeneration and Regeneration of the Nervous System* [7].

histiocytes of mesodermal origin as opposed to the epithelial origin of "classical" glia. Regarding microglia, he stated: "Since it is of different ancestry and its characteristics differ from those of the nerve cells (first element) and the neuroglial astrocytes (second element) [containing astrocytes and oligodendrocytes], the microglia constitutes the *true* third element of the central nervous system" [15].

However, there was still much debate on the existence of oligodendroglia as a distinct CNS cell type, due in part to the difficulty involved in staining these cells. In fact, Cajal was unable to produce an effective and reproducible stain, leading him to dismiss these cells altogether as a true class of glial cells and to declare that the "third element" was made up exclusively of microglia. Given Cajal's enormous influence, his dismissal was perhaps just as important as any staining difficulty with respect to the further characterization

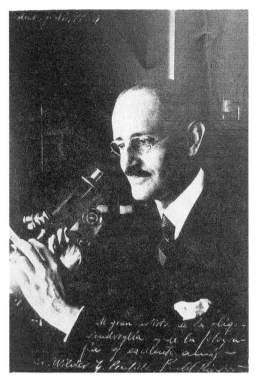

FIG. 3.5 Pío del Río-Hortega (1882–1945). Disciple of Cajal who worked with Penfield to co-discover oligodendroglial cells. As seen with a time exposure photograph taken from Wilder Penfield's simple box camera. Río-Hortega's inscription reads, "Al gran artista de la oligodendroglia y de la fotografía y excelente amigo—Wilder G. Penfield." ("To the great artist of oligodendroglia and of photography and excellent friend—Wilder G. Penfield"). *(Reproduced with permission from Gill AS, Binder DK. Wilder Penfield, Pío del Río-Hortega, and the discovery of oligodendroglia. Neurosurgery 2007;60(5):940–48.)*

of oligodendroglia. This put a strain on the relationship between Cajal and Río-Hortega. On Penfield's arrival in Spain, there had been no resolution to this debate (Fig. 3.6).

Penfield's description of oligodendroglia

Penfield noted that before the method of Río-Hortega, oligodendroglia were very difficult to stain completely. The first to stain oligodendroglial cells was the Scottish investigator William Ford Robertson (1867–1923) who employed a platinum method to describe cells that he termed *mesoglia* [16,17]. However, in his term *mesoglia*, he had just described a group of cells he believed to be of mesodermal origin. Penfield went back to examine an original preparation of Robertson and compared it with sections stained by Río-Hortega's method. He was able to verify that the "mesoglia" of Robertson was indeed identical to

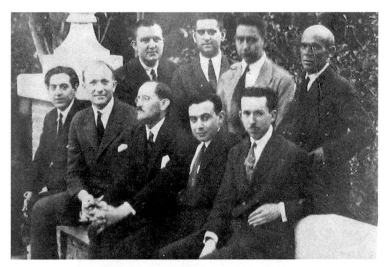

FIG. 3.6 Penfield (lower row, second from left) and Río-Hortega (lower row, center) in Spain with colleagues, 1924. *(Reproduced with permission from Gill AS, Binder DK. Wilder Penfield, Pío del Río-Hortega, and the discovery of oligodendroglia. Neurosurgery 2007;60(5):940–48.)*

the "oligodendroglia" of Río-Hortega. Based on this, Penfield suggested that the term "mesoglia" be abandoned.

Penfield then learned the method of Río-Hortega for staining oligodendroglial cells and added his modifications. Using the "ammoniacal silver carbonate" method of Río-Hortega, originally developed by Achúcarro [18], the results were variable. In 1924, Penfield reported on his modifications to the method and used it to stain oligodendroglia in the CNS of rabbits.

The remainder of the staining procedure consisted of washing, toning, fixing, dehydrating, and clearing the specimen. Toning, originally described by Cajal, consisted of substituting gold for silver. With his modifications, Penfield had finally succeeded in developing a reliable stain for oligodendroglia. Don Pío, having been shown Penfield's exceptional slides, remarked, *"Casi mejor que yo"* (almost better than I could do). Penfield later reminisced that he "might have laughed at his use of the word 'almost,'" but that "he could expect no higher praise" [3].

Río-Hortega then asked Penfield to publish his results confirming oligodendroglia as the remaining cell type of the "third element." Penfield studied and drew many of the oligodendroglia that he stained (Fig. 3.7). While noting that neuroglia and oligodendroglia both possessed "the asteroid body with expansions, centrosome and Golgi apparatus of similar appearance" [19], he nevertheless was able to distinguish many characteristics of oligodendroglia. He noted that oligodendroglial nuclei are larger than those of microglia but smaller than those of neuroglia. He also commented on the ability to distinguish neuroglia from oligodendroglia by the presence of "sucker feet" (modern-day "vascular

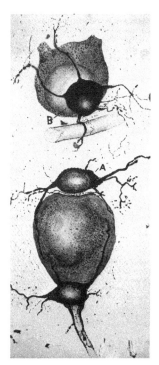

FIG. 3.7 Penfield's original drawing of perineuronal and perivascular oligodendroglia. *(Reproduced with permission from Penfield W. Oligodendroglia and its relation to classical neuroglia. Brain 1924;47:430–52.)*

endfeet") on the former group of cells [19]. Penfield also stated that with his improved methods he could get a better view of the oligodendroglial cell cytoplasm, showing that the "expansions" of cytoplasm were directed along the length of the "neuron cable system" (*i.e.* along white matter tracts) (Fig. 3.8). In addition to studying white matter oligodendroglia (termed "interfascicular glia" by Río-Hortega), Penfield carefully described oligodendroglia in gray matter as well. Penfield clearly showed that "perineuronal satellites" included *both* oligodendroglia and microglia. Similarly, he showed that "perivascular satellites" could also be either oligodendroglia or microglia. Critically, he noted that while the cell bodies of these two types of perivascular satellites were "applied closely to the blood-vessel," neither one was like neuroglia in this respect: With neuroglia, it was the "neuroglia expansions that are applied to the neuron and vessel." Interestingly, he may have simultaneously underestimated neuroglia and overestimated neurons in claiming that "oligodendroglia forms by far the most numerous group of cells in the central nervous system, after nerve cells" [19].

In 1924, Wilder Penfield published his work from *La Residencia* in a seminal article in the journal *Brain, Oligodendroglia and its relation to classical*

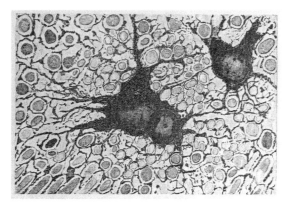

FIG. 3.8   Penfield's drawing depicting oligodendroglial expansions encircling myelin sheaths in the CNS of a rabbit. *(Reproduced with permission from Penfield W. Oligodendroglia and its relation to classical neuroglia, Brain 1924;47:430–52.)*

neuroglia [19]. In this article, he paid homage to his mentors Cajal and Río-Hortega:

> *In spite of untiring study of the central nervous system which has demonstrated the intricate morphology of neurones and neuroglia, a very numerous body of small cells (the third element of Cajal) continued to be refractory to staining methods... The brilliant studies of Del Río-Hortega show that these cells possess complicated expansions. By demonstrating their detailed structure, he was able to show that they fall into two groups, differing in form and function. One group, which he chose to denominate microglia, is of mesodermal origin, and the other, oligodendroglia, composing the more numerous portion of the cells, he believes to be of ectodermal origin [19].*

In this historic publication, Penfield summarized his work along with the work of Cajal and Río-Hortega in formulating an overall classification of the interstitial cells of the nervous system (Table 3.2). This gross classification has changed remarkably little since.

Glial alterations in neurological disease: Early concepts

Following developments in the concepts of neuroglia, neuropathologists started to recognize glial alterations in tissues in patients with neurological diseases. Carl Frommann (1831–92) found changes in glial cell morphology in the vicinity of demyelinating plaques [20]. Andriezen indicated that astrocytes "exhibit a morbid hypertrophy in pathological conditions" [21]. Franz Nissl (1860–1919) described two pathological cell types: *Stäbchenzellen* (rod cells), which appeared in demented patients' brains; and *Körnerzellen* (granule cells) or *Gitterzellen* (lattice cells) which were associated with disruption of the blood-brain barrier [22,23]. Alois Alzheimer (1864–1915) described an ameboid change in glial

TABLE 3.2 Penfield's formulation of the interstitial cells of the central nervous system.

Interstitial cells	In white matter	In gray matter
(1) Neuroglia, classical (ectodermal)	Fibrous	Protoplasmic
(2) Oligodendroglia (probably ectodermal)	Interfascicular	Perineuronal (satellite)
(3) Microglia (probably mesodermal)	Present (no subdivision)	Present and numerous (no subdivision)

Reproduced with permission from Penfield W. Oligodendroglia and its relation to classical neuroglia. Brain 1924;47:430–52.

cells in response to acute and chronic neurologic diseases, such as epilepsy, syphilis, and the disease that bears his name [24]. Nicolás Achúcarro, a Basque-born psychiatrist and neurohistologist who was a colleague and alumnus of Cajal, advanced the idea that dysfunction of neuroglia may itself produce brain diseases [25]. Critically for epilepsy and brain injury, the role of astrocytes in glial scar formation was recognized by Cajal, Río Hortega, and Penfield in the 1920s [26]. Cajal's later career (from 1903 through his death in 1934) was devoted largely to the investigation of pathological processes within the nervous system. This work was summarized in the classic of neuroscience *Degeneration and Regeneration of the Nervous System* [7].

From neurocytology to neuropathology: Toward understanding of the cicatrix

When he initially used Río-Hortega's stains, before leaving for Madrid, Penfield explained the results were, "very exciting, but also very confusing. What I saw was difficult to interpret" [3]. In a short 6 months in Madrid, not only did Penfield perfect a specific stain for oligodendroglia and describe this "third element" in the seminal 1924 *Brain* paper, but with Río-Hortega also moved from "pure" neuroscience to neuropathology in studying the reaction of glial cells to injury. In an article entitled "Cerebral cicatrix: the reaction of neuroglia and microglia to brain wounds" [26], they provide several observations regarding cellular changes following simple stab wounds:

> *The formation of a simple cicatrix in the brain presents the following stages: The first cellular change is observed in microglia cells which begin their phagocytic activity early and continue it for a long period. Later, the neuroglia astrocytes about the wound become swollen and those closest to the area of destruction or to obliterated vessels undergo clasmatodendrosis. There follows rapid amitotic*

division of the other astrocytes and the cells then become fibrous and arrange themselves typically in a radial fashion about the wound. Most of their expansions, and particularly the robust ones, are arranged like the spokes of a wheel with the site of the former stab as the hub...A connective tissue core forms at the center, connective-tissue collagen fibrils are laid down and the wound contracts [26].

It is noteworthy that their basic idea of these injury stages and the formation of the "cicatrix" (contracting scar) are essentially correct. Compare, for example, a modern neuropathology textbook:

In regions of tissue damage hematogenous monocytes infiltrate the CNS and phagocytose dead cells and necrotic debris. Swelling of astrocytes is a relatively rapid response. With time, reactive astrocytes proliferate and insinuate long cytoplasmic processes into the adjacent brain parenchyma, which appear as fibrils in appropriately stained preparations [27].

Others have recently verified "clasmatodendrosis," their term for the loss of distal astrocytic processes, in degenerative disorders such as Alzheimer's disease [28–30]. Although the details of gliosis and microglial response were not complete, the numerous observations and conjectures put forth by Río-Hortega and Penfield in this single publication are astonishing. Cerebral cicatrix [26] was intended by Penfield to be a combined publication with his 1924 *Brain* manuscript. The latter manuscript was to be a combined publication with the former. However, "Pío procrastinated. This was his old-time enemy. I could not get our results into print for three years, not until 1927" [3].

In 1927, back at the New York-Presbyterian Hospital, along with his research associate William V. Cone (Fig. 3.9), Penfield decided to write a "textbook on the general principles of neuropathology without describing specific diseases" [3]. (Cone was a remarkably astute innovator and scholar whom, if not for his reluctance to write papers, would undoubtedly be widely known to every modern neurosurgeon [31].) Penfield thought that moving beyond a simple description of various diseases to a mechanistic description of disease pathophysiology was an essential step in the eventual treatment of various neurological diseases. However, Penfield "realized, far too often, that someone else, somewhere in the world, could write a better chapter. I wrote to several to see if they would do a chapter for us. I was surprised when the invitations were readily accepted since my name carried no prestige as editor" [3]. Numerous sources [2,32–34] belie this self-effacing claim: Penfield was widely known and respected, even in 1927, by many of the most eminent scientists of the day. In any event, all of his requests to contribute to *Cytology and Cellular Pathology of the Nervous System* were accepted, save for Cajal who "alone refused, saying he had advancing arteriosclerosis, the histologist's way of describing old age" [3]. Río-Hortega also gave Penfield pause, for he had a habit of not responding to letters and telegrams. Penfield describes bombarding Río-Hortega "with letters and finally, received a telegram from him followed by a letter. 'Of course, I will write for your book. How could you think otherwise'" [3].

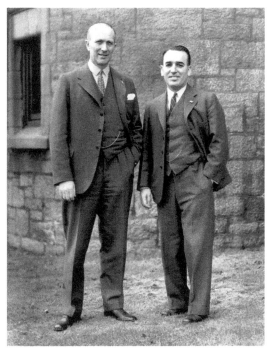

FIG. 3.9 Penfield and William V. Cone (1897–1959) outside the Royal Victoria Hospital, Montreal (c.1932). *(Reproduced with permission from Gill AS, Binder DK. Wilder Penfield, Pío del Río-Hortega, and the discovery of oligodendroglia. Neurosurgery 2007;60(5):940–48.)*

Cytology, dedicated to Cajal, was finally published in 1932 with 26 eminent contributors. It proved to be an instant and influential success. It was the first time written on neuropathology from a basic science perspective, a common staple of many pathology texts written today both for graduate and medical study. Penfield describes the reaction he received after the first edition went out of print:

When, eventually, the first edition of this reference book went out of print, I received letters of inquiry from all over the world. But I was too busy making clinical use of what I had learned to undertake a second edition. At long last, in 1965, Hafner, New York, reprinted it without change [3].

For such a text to be reprinted in original form more than 30 years after its first publication is a testament to its lasting influence.

Penfield credits the time he spent in Europe, specifically in Madrid, with providing him the "keys to understanding" [3]. At a time when glial cells were just being described and differentiated by Río-Hortega and himself, Penfield immediately studied their reaction to injury and their potential role in epilepsy. In his autobiography *No Man Alone*, he stated, "if one desired to throw new light on the effect of disease, or injury, and on the process of healing in the brain, the best hope lay in the study of the nonnervous cells, using Hortega's little-tried methods" [3]. More than 80 years after this statement was made, recent evidence is accumulating for a critical glial contribution to epilepsy [6,35,36].

Penfield was humble in acknowledging his mentors. He credited Sherrington with influencing his scientific thinking "more than anyone else," saying "I looked through his eyes and came to realize that here in the nervous system was the great unexplored field—the undiscovered country in which the mystery of the mind of man might someday be explained" [3]. In the obituary he wrote for Río-Hortega in 1945, Penfield makes no mention of his role in the authentication of oligodendroglia or the elucidation of microglia, giving full credit to Río-Hortega [37].

Penfield and Foerster: Toward neuropathology of posttraumatic epilepsy

Penfield's experience in Spain grounded him in state-of-the-art neurocytology and, as mentioned above, he had already applied this knowledge to the study of cellular response to injury in his 1927 paper with Río-Hortega *Cerebral cicatrix: the reaction of neuroglia and microglia to brain wounds* [26]. Río-Hortega and Penfield laid down a plausible neuropathological underpinning of posttraumatic epilepsy. Penfield hypothesized that the "meningocerebral cicatrix" caused the "discharging lesion" referred to by Hughlings Jackson. In a follow-up publication the same year (1927), Penfield further discussed *the mechanism of cicatricial contraction in the brain* [38]. In it, he states a key role for astrocytes:

> *The structural connection between vessels and nervous tissue is by means of the neuroglia astrocytes...the octopus-like astrocytes, therefore, hold the manifold structures of the nervous system within their tentacles, and are attached to pia and vascular tree by specialized expansions...for the sake of convenience in the discussion which follows, it will be referred to as the vaso-astral framework" [38].*

He goes on to state the primacy of changes in this vaso-astral framework as causative of the "meningocerebral cicatrix," which forms "when the pia mater is injured and cerebral tissue exposed." Penfield had been able to use Cajal's gold chloride-sublimate method to stain astrocytes selectively (Fig. 3.10).

Penfield described that after injury, "astrocyte expansions are capable of hypertrophy and elongation as shown by their marked tortuosity" (a clear description of what we would call today reactive astrocytosis) (Fig. 3.11). He further conjectured that the pial-based scar from a penetrating brain injury thus exerts "mechanical traction" on the subjacent brain tissue.

Penfield held that "just as connective tissue scars elsewhere in the body tend to contract, so contraction occurs in the brain" thereby exacerbating the mechanical traction exerted by the cicatrix. Interestingly, Penfield adduced evidence from Foerster who sent him pneumoencephalogram images illustrating

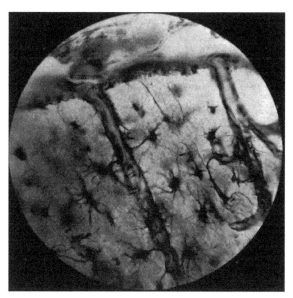

FIG. 3.10 Fibrous astrocytes about vessels entering cortex; normal. G.C.S. (gold chloride sublimate) stain, 326× magnification. *(Reproduced with permission from Penfield W. The mechanism of cicatricial contraction in the brain. Brain 1927;1:499–517.)*

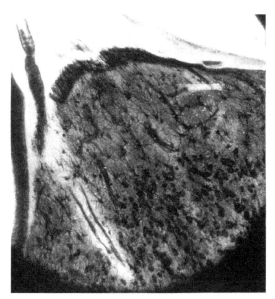

FIG. 3.11 Superficial pial adhesion near brain injury. The pia-arachnoid is unstained. Note hypertrophy of zonal glia and alignment of astrocytes below toward the pull. G.C.S. (gold chloride sublimate) stain, 184× magnification. *(Reproduced with permission from Penfield W. The mechanism of cicatricial contraction in the brain. Brain 1927;1:499–517.)*

the "wandering" of the ventricles to the side of the lesion (presumably reflecting the mechanical traction on more compliant brain structures) [38]. These considerations lead to the therapeutic conclusion that

> *the slow contraction of such a scar, continuing as it does for years, must produce a constant irritation which may well be the starting point for a nervous discharge resulting in Jacksonian epilepsy. Clean excision of such a cicatrix should convert a contracting scar into a fluid-filled space and relieve the remainder of the brain from abnormal traction [38].*

In 1928, Penfield had another experience that would inaugurate the first studies of the neuropathology of posttraumatic epilepsy in particular: He went to visit Otfrid Foerster in Breslau (Chapter 1). Per Pasteur's maxim "Chance favors a prepared mind," Penfield was ideally prepared with his neurohistological background and interest in posttraumatic epilepsy to get the most out of the visit to Foerster [39]. Together for that short time, they (1) conducted the first systematic histological study of posttraumatic epilepsy; (2) formulated a testable hypothesis of its etiology; and (3) developed a therapeutic rationale for replacing an epileptogenic meningocerebral cicatrix with a clean surgical wound [40]. Pathological examination of the posttraumatic scars revealed fibrous bands projecting inwards from the meningeal surface containing both blood vessels and collagenous fibers [41]. Foerster had observed that intraoperative seizures in his awake patients could be elicited by electrical stimulation near the meningocerebral cicatrix or by gentle traction on the cicatrix itself. Based on these observations, both Penfield and Foerster advocated radical but clean excision of the scar down to the ventricle [41].

Their joint report in 1930, *The structural basis of traumatic epilepsy and results of radical operation*, constitutes the first true histopathological study of posttraumatic epilepsy [41] (Fig. 3.12).

JULY, 1930.

BRAIN.

PART 2, VOL. 53.

THE STRUCTURAL BASIS OF TRAUMATIC EPILEPSY
AND RESULTS OF RADICAL OPERATION.[1]

BY O. FOERSTER,
Breslau,

AND

WILDER PENFIELD,
Montreal.

FIG. 3.12   Seminal 1930 publication by Foerster and Penfield demonstrating first pathological studies of PTE tissue and the results of extirpation of cortical scars. *(Reproduced with permission from Foerster O, Penfield W. The structural basis of traumatic epilepsy and results of radical operation. Brain 1930;53:99–119.)*

In this manuscript, they report seven cases of PTE examined with preoperative pneumoencephalography, treated surgically with intraoperative cortical stimulation, and then gross and microscopic pathological observation of resected tissue. Case #1 is a good example of their approach. This patient sustained a left parietal gunshot wound in 1914 with subsequent Jacksonian epilepsy starting on the right side in 1920 (*i.e.* 6 years after the trauma). Pneumoencephalography in 1925 showed some enlargement of the left lateral ventricle and a displacement of both lateral and third ventricles toward the side of the lesion (Fig. 3.13). In 1925, a large left parietal craniotomy was performed and the dura mater was found to be densely adherent to an underlying brain scar and cyst. Electrical stimulation revealed that the lesion lay just posterior to the motor area for the fingers. A wide excision was carried out as indicated by the broken line in Fig. 3.14.

The gross specimen "showed considerable thickening of the dura" and "a bit of bone was embedded in the cicatrix and bands of fibrous tissue could be seen passing downwards into the brain" (Fig. 3.15). Microscopic examination revealed connective tissue entering the brain scar (Fig. 3.16). This included both collagen fibers and blood vessels. Deeper in the brain, neuroglia fibers were also found "lying in parallel lines, pointing upwards towards the meningocerebral adhesion" (Fig. 3.17).

After removal of the meningocerebral cicatrix, this patient (Case 1) "made a good recovery and in the five years following the operation up to the time when last heard of he was quite free from convulsive seizures" [41]. The remainder

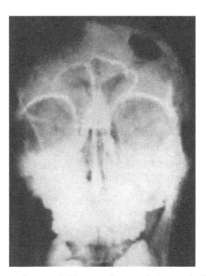

FIG. 3.13 Encephalogram (brow up) 11 years after gunshot wound of the left parietal region. Cranial defect is shown and lateral ventricles are pulled toward it. Case 1 from Foerster and Penfield 1930. *(Reproduced with permission from Foerster O, Penfield W. The structural basis of traumatic epilepsy and results of radical operation. Brain 1930;53:99–119.)*

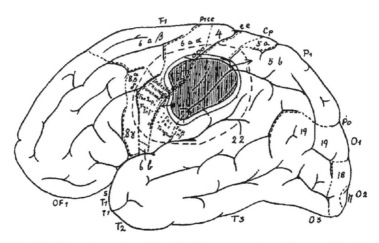

FIG. 3.14 Shaded area shows the position of the lesion at operation and the second line the extent of operative removal. Case 1 from Foerster and Penfield 1930. *(Reproduced with permission from Foerster O, Penfield W. The structural basis of traumatic epilepsy and results of radical operation. Brain 1930;53:99–119.)*

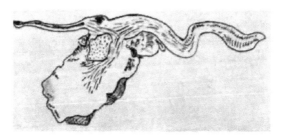

FIG. 3.15 Cross-section of cicatrix attached to thickened dura. Case 1 from Foerster and Penfield 1930. *(Reproduced with permission from Foerster O, Penfield W. The structural basis of traumatic epilepsy and results of radical operation. Brain 1930;53:99–119.)*

of this seminal manuscript describes six other similar cases of PTE treated by "radical operation" with generally excellent results and similar neuropathological findings.

Interestingly, after Penfield's visit, the Rockefeller Foundation supported the establishment of a neurological institute under Foerster's direction in Breslau. Foerster continued his work there through Weimar Germany and the rise of National Socialism (Nazism). Despite his worldwide eminence, his ties to Russia (having treated Lenin) and the United States (being funded by the Rockefeller Foundation) led to great suspicion among the authorities in Nazi Germany, so much so that he was deprived of his extraordinary professorship in 1934 and relieved of the function of a university professor in 1938 [42]. Foerster succumbed to tuberculosis in Breslau in 1941 during the height of World War II. Ironically, an American bomb destroyed the Foerster Neurological Institute [39].

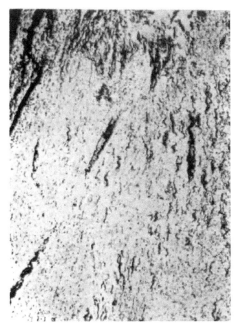

FIG. 3.16 Connective tissue and vessels entering the brain scar in parallel strands. Silver carbonate collagen stain. Case 1 from Foerster and Penfield 1930. *(Reproduced with permission from Foerster O, Penfield W. The structural basis of traumatic epilepsy and results of radical operation. Brain 1930;53:99–119.)*

Penfield's other contributions

After the visit to Breslau, Penfield arrived in Montreal in November 1928 and proceeded to operate with his surgical partner (William Cone, Fig. 3.9) using the Foerster method (awake craniotomy and brain mapping). Penfield and his colleagues subsequently made seminal contributions to the mapping of the intact human brain, many contributions to epilepsy surgery, and the founding of the Montreal Neurological Institute (MNI) in September 1934 [2,32–34,43–45]. Under Penfield's direction, the MNI made key developments in both human brain mapping and a modern anatomical and neurophysiological approach to epilepsy [45–47]. As an Oslerian "medico-chirurgical neurologist" [33], Penfield indeed embodied the ultimate combination of neuroscientist and neurosurgeon. When comparing physician investigators to pure scientists, Penfield offers advice that is as true today as it was then: "We have our practical purposes. We must select our weapons and plan our research with the patient and his unique problems in mind" [3].

Although epilepsy remained Penfield's "great teacher" [3], and despite Penfield's and the MNI's many contributions, what was still lacking included: (1) adequate imaging to assess structural lesions of the brain noninvasively to correlate with subsequent electrophysiology; and (2) a detailed pathophysiological

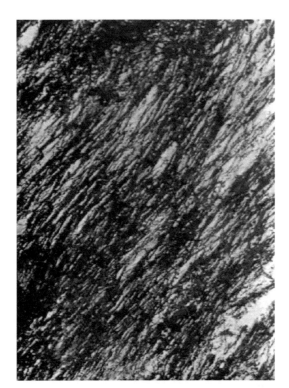

FIG. 3.17 Parallel neuroglia fibers oriented in the direction of the cicatricial pull. Silver carbonate astrocyte stain, Hortega. Case 1 from Foerster and Penfield 1930. *(Reproduced with permission from Foerster O, Penfield W. The structural basis of traumatic epilepsy and results of radical operation, Brain 1930;53:99–119.)*

understanding of the "discharging lesion." The first would have to await modern computed tomography (CT) and magnetic resonance imaging (MRI) structural and functional imaging; the second is the topic of much of this book and is still poorly understood. In 1961, Penfield himself indicated that

> *Through trauma the brain may be injured by contusion, laceration, compression, and it is well known that these insults may result in epilepsy after a 'silent period of strange ripening.' That period lasts for months or years, but these insults produce epilepsy in the case of one individual and not in the case of another. When there is widespread injury of a man's brain, epileptic discharge may develop in one area of that brain and not in another. Our attention should therefore be directed toward the discovery of this mysterious difference. What happens during the ripening period of A who develops fits? What influences A adversely? Or, perhaps, what influences B favorably? It is not enough to describe the destruction or sclerotic alteration of neurons, the phagocytosis carried out by microglia, the disappearance of oligodendroglia, and multiplication and fibrillation of astrocytes [48].*

Indeed, much of the modern effort toward understanding the pathophysiology of PTE described in this book is to undercover the mechanisms operative during Penfield's "silent period of strange ripening" (*i.e.* posttraumatic epileptogenesis).

Toward more modern histopathology: TBI to PTE?

Traumatic brain injury (TBI) results when force transmitted to the head results in neuropathological damage. Epidemiological studies have indicated a much higher incidence of PTE after severe TBI, particularly after penetrating injuries (Chapter 2). However, the exact type and nature of the pathological changes that underpin the development of PTE after TBI as opposed to TBI that does not lead to PTE remain unclear and are the topic of the remainder of this book. Animal studies (summarized later in this book) may ultimately be able to distinguish the cascade of neuropathological and neurophysiological changes that lead to PTE as distinct from the neuropathology of TBI *per se*.

TBI can be categorized in multiple ways to aid in correlation to the development of PTE [49]. The severity of the injury is most commonly quantified by the GCS (Glasgow Coma Scale) score (Table 3.3). TBIs can also be categorized as focal versus diffuse injuries. Focal injuries include mass lesions such as contusions, subdural hematomas, epidural hematomas, intraparenchymal hemorrhages, and depressed skull fractures. Diffuse injuries include diffuse axonal injury (DAI, shearing of axons) and hypoxic-ischemic injury. Third categorization is primary versus secondary injury. Primary injuries result from the direct mechanical forces deforming and damaging brain tissue, including forces such as acceleration, deceleration, rotational forces, blast injury, blunt impact, and penetrating impact. Secondary injuries results from a cascade of

TABLE 3.3 Glasgow Coma Scale.

Standard Glasgow Coma Scale score

Eye opening	Best verbal response	Best motor response
4: spontaneous	5: oriented	6: obeys commands
3: to speech	4: confused	5: localizes
2: to pain	3: inappropriate words	4: withdraws
1: none	2: incomprehensible sounds	3: abnormal flexion
	1: none	2: extension
		1: none

Total GCS score: 3–15

Reproduced with permission from McKee AC, Daneshvar DH. The neuropathology of traumatic brain injury. In: Grafman J, Salazar AM, Editors. Traumatic brain injury. Elsevier; 2015. p. 45–66.

potentially reversible secondary events such as ischemic and hypoxic damage, cerebral edema, elevated intracranial pressure, hydrocephalus, infection, and neuroinflammation [49].

It is clear based on the epidemiological studies (Chapter 2) that severity of the injury and particularly the presence of penetrating injury through the dura are the factors most strongly predisposing to the subsequent development of PTE. However, the central difficulty of understanding the neuropathology of PTE in modern neuropathological terms is that most patients subjected to TBI do not develop epilepsy and epilepsy develops delayed from the actual TBI. Thus, PTE may develop many months to many years after the TBI, and the cascade of contributory events over that prolonged period is poorly understood. Thus, while we have a very good modern understanding of the neuropathology of various types of TBI [49], the actual neuropathological factors responsible for the transition to PTE are much less clear. It is hoped that a detailed study of appropriate neuropathological specimens resected from patients with PTE may be feasible in the modern era (as pioneered by Foerster and Penfield) but with more modern molecular and cellular approaches. Remarkably, however, no modern studies of human PTE neuropathology (as distinct from TBI neuropathology) have been published. It is hoped that the study of human pathological specimens resected from patients with PTE can be reinvigorated in a cellular and molecular context and together with study of appropriate TBI animal models with and without PTE help to shed light on the key neuropathological underpinnings of PTE.

References

[1] Gill AS, Binder DK. Wilder Penfield, Pío del Río-Hortega, and the discovery of oligodendroglia. Neurosurgery 2007;60(5):940–8.

[2] Preul MC, Feindel W. Origins of Wilder Penfield's surgical technique: the role of the "Cushing ritual" and influences from the European experience. J Neurosurg 1991;75:812–20.

[3] Penfield W. No man alone: a neurosurgeon's life. Boston, MA: Little, Brown and Company; 1977.

[4] Penfield W. The career of Ramón y Cajal. Arch Neurol Psychiatry 1926;16:213–20.

[5] Shepherd GM. Foundations of the neuron doctrine. New York: Oxford University Press; 1991. p. 338. ix.

[6] Hubbard JA, Binder DK. Astrocytes and epilepsy. Amsterdam: Elsevier/Academic Press; 2016.

[7] Ramón y Cajal S. Degeneration and regeneration of the nervous system. London: Oxford University Press; 1928.

[8] Golgi C. Sulla fina anatomia degli organi centrali del sistema nervoso. Milano: Ulrico Hoepli; 1885. p. 215.

[9] Golgi C. Sur l' anatomia microscopique des organes centraux su Systéme nerveux. Arch Ital Biol 1886;7:15–47.

[10] Ramón y Cajal S. Contribucion al conocimiento de la neuroglia del cerebro humano. Trab Lab Inv Biol 1913;11:215–315.

[11] Ramón y Cajal S. Sobre un nuevo proceder de impregnacion de la neuroglia y sus resultados en los centros nerviosis del hombre y animales. Trab Lab Inv Biol 1913;11:219–37.

[12] Del Río-Hortega P. Noticia de un nuevo y facil metodo para la coloracion de la neuroglia y del tejido conjunctivo. Trab Lab Inv Biol 1918;15:367–78.

[13] Tremblay ME, et al. From the Cajal alumni Achúcarro and Río-Hortega to the rediscovery of never-resting microglia. Front Neuroanat 2015;9:45.

[14] Rezaie P, Male D. Mesoglia & microglia—a historical review of the concept of mononuclear phagocytes within the central nervous system. J Hist Neurosci 2002;11:325–74.

[15] Del Río-Hortega P. Microglia. In: Penfield W, editor. Cytology and cellular pathology of the nervous system. New York: Hafner; 1932. p. 483–534.

[16] Robertson WF. The normal histology and pathology of the neuroglia (in relation specially to mental diseases). J Ment Sci 1897;43:733–52.

[17] Robertson WF. A microscopic demonstration of the normal and pathological history of mesoglia cells. J Ment Sci 1900;46:724.

[18] Achúcarro N. Nuevo método para el estudio de la neuroglia y del tejido conjuntivo. Bol Soc Esp Biol 1911;1:139–41.

[19] Penfield W. Oligodendroglia and its relation to classical neuroglia. Brain 1924;47:430–52.

[20] Frommann C. Untersuchung über die Gewebsveränderungen bei der Multiplen Sklerose des Gehirns. Jena: Gustav Fischer; 1878.

[21] Andriezen WL. The neuroglia elements of the brain. Br Med J 1893;2:227–30.

[22] Nissl F. Über einigen Beziehungen zur Nervenzellenerkrankungen und gliosen Erscheinungen bei verschiedene Psychosen. Arch Psychiatrie 1899;32:656–76.

[23] Nissl F. Die Histopathologie der paralytischen Rindenerkrankung. In: Nissl F, editor. Histologische und histopathologische Arbeiten über die Grosshirnrinde mit besonderer Berücksichtigung der pathologischen Anatomie der Geisteskrankheiten, vol. 1. Jena: Gustav Fischer; 1904.

[24] Alzheimer A. Beiträge zur Kenntnis der pathologischen Neuroglia und ihrer Beziehungen zu den Abbauvorgängen im Nervengewebe. In: Nissl F, Alzheimer A, editors. Histologische und histopathologische Arbeiten über die Grosshirnrinde mit besonderer Berücksichtigung der pathologischen Anatomie der Geisteskrankheiten. Jena: Gustav Fischer; 1910. p. 401–562.

[25] Achúcarro N. Notas sobra la estructura y funciones de la neuroglía y en particular de la neuroglía de la corteza cerebral humana. Trab Lab Invest Biol Univ Madrid 1913;3:1–31.

[26] Del Río-Hortega P, Penfield WG. Cerebral cicatrix: the reaction of neuroglia and microglia to brain wounds. Bull Johns Hopkins Hosp 1927;41:278–303.

[27] Ellison D, Love S. Neuropathology. London: Mosby International Ltd; 1998.

[28] Sahlas DJ, Bilbao JM, Swartz RH, Black SE. Clasmatodendrosis correlating with periventricular hyperintensity in mixed dementia. Ann Neurol 2002;52(3):378–81.

[29] Hulse RE, et al. Astrocytic clasmatodendrosis in hippocampal organ culture. Glia 2001;33(2):169–79.

[30] Tomimoto H, et al. Alterations of the blood-brain barrier and glial cells in white-matter lesions in cerebrovascular and Alzheimer's disease patients. Stroke 1996;27(11):2069–74.

[31] Preul MC, et al. Neurosurgeon as innovator: William V. Cone (1897-1959). J Neurosurg 1993;79:619–31.

[32] Feindel W. Harvey Cushing's Canadian connections. Neurosurgery 2003;52:198–208.

[33] Feindel W. Osler and the "medico-chirurgical neurologists": Horsley, Cushing, and Penfield. J Neurosurg 2003;99:188–99.

[34] Preul MC, Feindel W. "the art is long and the life short": the letters of Wilder Penfield and Harvey Cushing. J Neurosurg 2001;95:148–61.

[35] Binder DK, Steinhäuser C. Functional changes in astroglial cells in epilepsy. Glia 2006;54(5):358–68.

[36] Tian G-F, et al. An astrocytic basis of epilepsy. Nat Med 2005;11(9):973–81.

[37] Penfield W. Obituaries: Pío Del Río-Hortega, M.D. (1882-1945). Arch Neurol Psychiatry 1945;54:413–6.

[38] Penfield W. The mechanism of cicatricial contraction in the brain. Brain 1927;1:499–517.

[39] Penfield W. Lights in the great darkness: the 1971 Harvey Cushing oration. J Neurosurg 1971;35(4):377–83.

[40] Feindel W, Leblanc R, Villemure J-G. History of the surgical treatment of epilepsy. In: Greenblatt SH, Dagi TF, Epstein MH, editors. A history of neurosurgery in its scientific and professional contexts. Park Ridge, IL: American Association of Neurological Surgeons; 1997.

[41] Foerster O, Penfield W. The structural basis of traumatic epilepsy and results of radical operation. Brain 1930;53:99–119.

[42] Piotrowska N, Winkler PA. Otfrid Foerster, the great neurologist and neurosurgeon from Breslau (Wrocław): his influence on early neurosurgeons and legacy to present-day neurosurgery. J Neurosurg 2007;107(2):451–6.

[43] Almeida AN, Martinez V, Feindel W. The first case of invasive EEG monitoring for the surgical treatment of epilepsy: historical significance and context. Epilepsia 2005;46:1082–5.

[44] Feindel W. The Montreal Neurological Institute. J Neurosurg 1991;75:821–2.

[45] Leblanc R. Radical treatment: Wilder Penfield's life in neuroscience. Montreal: McGill-Queen's University Press; 2020.

[46] Penfield W, Boldrey E. Somatic motor and sensory representation in the cerebral cortex of man as studied by electrical stimulation. Brain 1937;60:389–443.

[47] Penfield W, Jasper H. Epilepsy and the functional anatomy of the human brain. Boston, MA: Little, Brown & Co.; 1954.

[48] Penfield W. Introduction (symposium on post-traumatic epilepsy). Epilepsia 1961;2:109–10.

[49] McKee AC, Daneshvar DH. The neuropathology of traumatic brain injury. In: Grafman J, Salazar AM, editors. Traumatic brain injury. Elsevier; 2015. p. 45–66.

Chapter 4

Clinical trials of agents to prevent posttraumatic epilepsy

Overview

Posttraumatic epilepsy (PTE) is theoretically preventable since PTE may follow traumatic brain injury (TBI) after months to years. This provides a potential "treatment window" to prevent posttraumatic epileptogenesis after TBI. There have been several clinical trials of antiepileptic drugs to try to prevent PTE. In this chapter, we review these trials in chronological order. Agents that have been tested include phenytoin, phenobarbital, carbamazepine, valproate, magnesium, and levetiracetam. None of these agents prevented the development of late seizures (PTE) after TBI. The absence of any effective antiepileptogenic agents against PTE should stimulate novel clinical trials based on new targets.

Vietnam prophylaxis program

The concept of PTE prophylaxis originated in the treatment of veterans of the Vietnam War [1,2]. The Vietnam prophylaxis program was regularly incorporated into head injuries. Rish and Caveness reported the results in 1973 [2]. The protocol was to receive 300–400 mg/day phenytoin (in 93% of patients), phenobarbital 96 mg/day (in 4% of patients), or both (in 3% of patients). Of 1614 Vietnam War veterans analyzed, 1136 (70%) received anticonvulsant therapy, 465 (29%) received no prophylactic regimen, and in 13 (1%) the presence or absence of a prophylactic regimen could not be determined [2]. The incidence of early seizures (within the first week postinjury) in the prophylactically treated group was 18/1136, or 1.6% compared to 17/465 or 3.7% within the untreated group. This difference, however, was not statistically significant. The authors concluded that "the prophylactic use of anticonvulsants in combat head injuries needs to be reconsidered" [2]. In addition, the overall similarity of incidence of PTE in Vietnam compared to prior wars (Chapter 2) provides no support for the efficacy of this specific prophylactic regime practiced in Vietnam War veterans.

Posttraumatic Epilepsy. https://doi.org/10.1016/B978-0-323-90099-7.00006-X

67

Carbamazepine study

In 1983, Glötzner and colleagues published a single study regarding seizure prevention by carbamazepine following severe TBI; 139 patients above 15 years of age with severe TBI were included in the study and were randomly divided into carbamazepine and placebo groups. Prophylaxis was started after the TBI and was continued for 1.5–2 years. Carbamazepine dosage was adjusted to achieve therapeutic serum levels. Carbamazepine was found to reduce early seizures (within the first week after TBI) but did not affect the incidence of late posttraumatic seizures [3].

Phenytoin studies

In 1983, Young et al. reported a prospective, double-blinded study of 179 head-injured adult patients treated with phenytoin or placebo for 18 months [4]. Patients received loading doses of phenytoin or placebo and drug levels were monitored. By the end of the study, 12.9% of treated patients and 10.8% of control patients had seizures. Thus, this study provided no evidence of benefit of phenytoin in seizure prevention.

In the same year, the same group reported a similar study on pediatric patients. Forty-one pediatric patients with head injuries were randomized into either phenytoin or placebo and followed for 18 months. The patients were parenterally administered phenytoin or placebo until oral doses could be tolerated. There was no significant difference in the percentage of children having seizures in the treated and placebo groups ($P = .25$) [5].

The most influential study of phenytoin prophylaxis of PTE was conducted by Nancy Temkin and colleagues in 1990 [6]; 404 patients with severe TBI were prospectively enrolled to receive either phenytoin ($n = 208$) or placebo ($n = 196$). An intravenous loading dose was given within 24 h of injury. Serum levels were assessed and drug levels were maintained in the high therapeutic range. Follow-up was continued for 2 years. This study found that between drug loading and day 7, 3.6% of patients assigned to phenytoin had seizures as compared with 14.2% of patients assigned to placebo ($P < .001$) (Fig. 4.1). At the end of year 2, the rates of seizures were 27.5% in the phenytoin group and 21.1% in the placebo group ($P > .2$) (Fig. 4.2). They concluded that phenytoin reduces early posttraumatic seizures but does not prevent late posttraumatic seizures (i.e. PTE).

A subsequent follow-up study by the same investigators evaluated side effects and mortality associated with the use of phenytoin for early posttraumatic seizure prophylaxis [7]. This was a secondary analysis of data obtained from the 404 patients from the original New England Journal of Medicine study [6]. In this follow-up study, the investigators found that phenytoin indeed reduces the incidence of early posttraumatic seizures without a significant increase in drug-related side effects, and there was no effect on mortality [7].

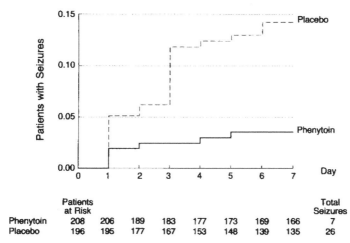

FIG. 4.1 Cumulative fraction of patients with early seizures (between drug loading and Day 7). The number of patients observed and at risk for seizures and the total number of seizures are shown at the bottom of the figure. The seizure rate was significantly lower in the phenytoin group ($P < .001$). *(Reproduced with permission from Temkin NR, et al. A randomized, double-blind study of phenytoin for the prevention of post-traumatic seizures. New Engl J Med 1990;323(8):497–502.)*

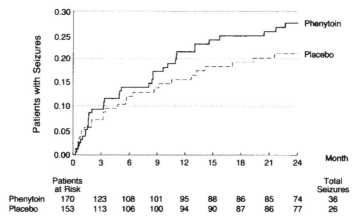

FIG. 4.2 Cumulative fraction of patients with late seizures (after Day 8). The number of patients at risk for seizures and the total number of seizures are shown at the bottom of the figure. The seizure rates were similar in the phenytoin and placebo groups. *(Reproduced with permission from Temkin NR, et al. A randomized, double-blind study of phenytoin for the prevention of post-traumatic seizures. New Engl J Med 1990;323(8):497–502.)*

Valproate study

In 1999, Temkin and colleagues published a randomized, double-blind, single-center clinical trial of valproate for the prevention of PTE [8]. This involved three treatment arms: (1) 1-week course of phenytoin; (2) 1-month course of valproate; and (3) 6-month course of valproate. Treatment began within 24h of injury. Follow-up was 2 years. They found similar rates of early seizures when using either valproate or phenytoin. The rates of late seizures did not differ among treatment groups. The authors concluded that valproate therapy shows no benefit in preventing late seizures [8].

Magnesium study

In 2007, Temkin *et al.* reported a double-blind trial of magnesium sulfate administration after TBI [9]; 499 patients aged 14 years or older admitted to a trauma center with moderate or severe TBI were randomly assigned one of two doses of magnesium or placebo within 8 h of injury and continuing for 5 days. The primary outcome was a composite of mortality, seizures, functional measures, and neuropsychological tests assessed up to 6 months after injury. The authors found that magnesium showed no significant positive effect on the composite primary outcome measure at the higher dose. Those randomly assigned magnesium at the lower dose did significantly worse than those assigned placebo. Furthermore, there was higher mortality with the higher magnesium dose than with placebo. They concluded that continuous infusions of magnesium for 5 days given to patients within 8 h of moderate or severe traumatic brain injury were not neuroprotective and might even have a negative effect in the treatment of significant head injury [9].

Levetiracetam studies

In 2010, Szaflarski *et al.* reported a prospective, single-center, randomized, single-blinded comparative trial of levetiracetam versus phenytoin in seizure prophylaxis after neurological injury [10]. Patients received intravenous (IV) loading with either levetiracetam or fosphenytoin followed by standard IV doses adjusted to maintain therapeutic serum levels. A total of 52 patients were randomized (levetiracetam, 34; phenytoin, 18). This study found a significant improvement in the Extended Glasgow Outcome Scale Score with lower disability at 6 months in patients receiving levetiracetam, but no difference in the occurrence of early or late posttraumatic seizures was observed between the groups (follow-up was to 6 months postinjury) [10].

In 2014, Gabriel *et al.* reported a single-center prospective cohort analysis of patients receiving levetiracetam or phenytoin after TBI [11]. Patients were then followed for 6 months for Extended Glasgow Outcome Scale Score and seizure outcomes. Nineteen patients were included in the final analysis. There was no difference in the occurrence of early or late posttraumatic seizures, and there was also no difference in the Extended Glasgow Outcome Scale Score [11].

The above levetiracetam studies were subsequently mentioned in two systematic reviews of the literature but without any change in the conclusion that levetiracetam is, like phenytoin, ineffective in preventing late posttraumatic seizures [12,13].

Perspective

Multiple review articles and metaanalyses summarizing the literature on prophylaxis for PTE have been published [14–23]. These articles concur that prophylactic antiepileptic drugs are effective in reducing early seizures, but no drug tested has been shown to prevent late seizures (PTE) after TBI. Chadwick (2000) concludes somewhat pessimistically that "Therefore, there seems no justification for the routine use of antiepileptic drugs in patients with severe head injuries. The pathway from severe head injury to posttraumatic epilepsy seems to be determined at the time of the injury and cannot thereafter be diverted by the clinician" [15]. Beghi (2003) is somewhat more optimistic in that he states "the identification of antiepileptogenic drugs should be made through interdisciplinary research and communication between clinical and basic scientists" [14]. Similarly, after all of the clinical trials that she pioneered, Nancy Temkin stated (2009) that "we need more laboratory work to better understand the process of epileptogenesis and to identify targets and therapies that might stop the process before epilepsy develops" [17]. It is the promise of the basic science of PTE as explored later in this book to identify new and much more promising targets for PTE to then translate into future clinical trials. The fact remains that entering the third decade of the 21st century still no drug has been found to be antiepileptogenic after TBI. This huge clinical gap should be ample stimulus for significant investment in new approaches, targets, and trials.

References

[1] Raymont V, et al. "Studying injured minds"—the Vietnam head injury study and 40 years of brain injury research. Front Neurol 2011;2:15.

[2] Rish BL, Caveness WF. Relation of prophylactic medication to the occurrence of early seizures following craniocerebral trauma. J Neurosurg 1973;38(2):155–8.

[3] Glötzner FL, et al. Seizure prevention using carbamazepine following severe brain injuries. Neurochirurgia (Stuttg) 1983;26(3):66–79.

[4] Young B, et al. Failure of prophylactically administered phenytoin to prevent late posttraumatic seizures. J Neurosurg 1983;58(2):236–41.

[5] Young B, et al. Failure of prophylactically administered phenytoin to prevent post-traumatic seizures in children. Childs Brain 1983;10(3):185–92.

[6] Temkin NR, et al. A randomized, double-blind study of phenytoin for the prevention of posttraumatic seizures. N Engl J Med 1990;323(8):497–502.

[7] Haltiner AM, et al. Side effects and mortality associated with use of phenytoin for early posttraumatic seizure prophylaxis. J Neurosurg 1999;91(4):588–92.

[8] Temkin NR, et al. Valproate therapy for prevention of posttraumatic seizures: a randomized trial. J Neurosurg 1999;91(4):593–600.

[9] Temkin NR, et al. Magnesium sulfate for neuroprotection after traumatic brain injury: a randomised controlled trial. Lancet Neurol 2007;6(1):29–38.

[10] Szaflarski JP, et al. Prospective, randomized, single-blinded comparative trial of intravenous levetiracetam versus phenytoin for seizure prophylaxis. Neurocrit Care 2010;12(2):165–72.

[11] Gabriel WM, Rowe AS. Long-term comparison of GOS-E scores in patients treated with phenytoin or levetiracetam for posttraumatic seizure prophylaxis after traumatic brain injury. Ann Pharmacother 2014;48(11):1440–4.

[12] Bakr A, Belli A. A systematic review of levetiracetam versus phenytoin in the prevention of late post-traumatic seizures and survey of UK neurosurgical prescribing practice of antiepileptic medication in acute traumatic brain injury. Br J Neurosurg 2018;32(3):237–44.

[13] Yang Y, et al. Levetiracetam versus phenytoin for seizure prophylaxis following traumatic brain injury: a systematic review and meta-analysis. CNS Drugs 2016;30(8):677–88.

[14] Beghi E. Overview of studies to prevent posttraumatic epilepsy. Epilepsia 2003;44(s10):21–6.

[15] Chadwick D. Seizures and epilepsy after traumatic brain injury. Lancet 2000;355(9201):334–6.

[16] Dunn LT, Foy PM. Anticonvulsant and antibiotic prophylaxis in head injury. Ann R Coll Surg Engl 1994;76(3):147–9.

[17] Temkin NR. Preventing and treating posttraumatic seizures: the human experience. Epilepsia 2009;50:10–3.

[18] Schierhout G, Roberts I. Prophylactic antiepileptic agents after head injury: a systematic review. J Neurol Neurosurg Psychiatry 1998;64(1):108–12.

[19] Teasell R, et al. Post-traumatic seizure disorder following acquired brain injury. Brain Inj 2007;21(2):201–14.

[20] D'Ambrosio R, Perucca E. Epilepsy after head injury. Curr Opin Neurol 2004;17(6):731–5.

[21] Christensen J. The epidemiology of posttraumatic epilepsy. Semin Neurol 2015;35(3):218–22.

[22] Chang BS, Lowenstein DH, Quality Standards Subcommittee of the American Academy of N. Practice parameter: antiepileptic drug prophylaxis in severe traumatic brain injury: report of the Quality Standards Subcommittee of the American Academy of Neurology. Neurology 2003;60(1):10–6.

[23] Kirmani BF, et al. Role of anticonvulsants in the management of posttraumatic epilepsy. Front Neurol 2016;7:32.

Chapter 5

Surgical treatment of posttraumatic epilepsy

Overview

In this chapter, we review the surgical treatment of posttraumatic epilepsy (PTE). Early neurosurgeons such as Foerster and Penfield (Chapters 1 and 3) had advocated radical excision of "meningocerebral cicatrices" down to the ventricle during awake craniotomies with intraoperative stimulation mapping. In this chapter, we start with this original concept and follow through the work of A. Earl Walker at Johns Hopkins and then summarize modern studies and case series of surgical treatment approaches and outcomes for PTE. An illustrative case example is presented demonstrating the potential surgical cure of PTE in selected cases.

Arthur Earl Walker

Following Penfield and Foerster's first foray into the neuropathology and surgical therapy of PTE in their 1930 publication [1] (Chapter 3), there was little progress in this field until the efforts of A. Earl Walker (Fig. 5.1).

Walker was born in 1907 in Winnipeg, Manitoba. He graduated from the University of Alberta then underwent training at Yale University and in Amsterdam and Brussels and then became an instructor of neurological surgery at the University of Chicago in 1937. During World War II, he worked as Chief of Neurology at Cushing General Hospital in Framingham, Massachusetts. From 1947 to 1972, he was a professor of neurological surgery at the Johns Hopkins Hospital.

Walker made numerous contributions to neurosurgery and neuroscience including: (1) In 1938, he published his monograph *The Primate Thalamus* [2]; (2) in 1942 he published two articles which would both lead to eponymous conditions bearing his name: *Dandy-Walker syndrome* (congenital atresia of the foramina of Luschka and Magendie) [3] and *Walker-Warburg syndrome* (lissencephaly) [4]; (3) In 1946, he demonstrated the convulsive effects of antibiotic agents on the cerebral cortex [5]; (4) In 1949, he published a monograph entitled *Posttraumatic Epilepsy* [6] (Fig. 5.2); (5) In 1951, he was the primary editor of *A History of Neurological Surgery* [7]; (6) Walker made contributions to neurosurgical education establishing the division of neurosurgery at Johns

Posttraumatic Epilepsy. https://doi.org/10.1016/B978-0-323-90099-7.00007-1

73

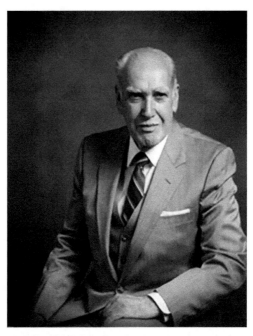

FIG. 5.1   Arthur Earl Walker (1907–95). Canadian-born American neurosurgeon. Known for detailed study of the primate thalamus, posttraumatic epilepsy, and the history of neurological surgery. Eponymously remembered for *Dandy-Walker syndrome* (congenital atresia of the foramina of Luschka and Magendie) and *Walker-Warburg syndrome* (lissencephaly).

Hopkins and the formal residency training program in neurosurgery; and (7) Walker served in national and international leadership positions (president of the American Association of Neurological Surgeons and the World Federation of Neurosurgical Societies).

Walker became interested in posttraumatic epilepsy during World War II. He and his colleagues made many contributions to the study of the epidemiology of PTE using military data from World War I, World War II, and the Korean War [8–13] (Chapter 2). In addition to studying PTE epidemiology, however, Walker also was directly involved in trying to advance the neuropathological understanding and surgical treatment of PTE. His experience in this regard is summarized in his monograph *Posttraumatic Epilepsy* from 1949 [6].

In this monograph, Walker first reviews what is known about the incidence of PTE. "In the latter part of November 1945, the Surgeon General of the United States Army designated Cushing General Hospital, Framingham, Massachusetts, as a center for the treatment of patients suffering from posttraumatic epilepsy… Much of the information in this discussion was acquired as the result of the author's experience in this center for posttraumatic epilepsy." So clearly it was the case that Walker, by dint of his appointment at Cushing General Hospital during World War II, became uniquely experienced in the treatment of World

POSTTRAUMATIC EPILEPSY

by

A. EARL WALKER, M.D.

Formerly, Professor of Neurological Surgery
University of Chicago, Chicago, Illinois
Now, Professor of Neurological Surgery
The Johns Hopkins University, Baltimore, Maryland

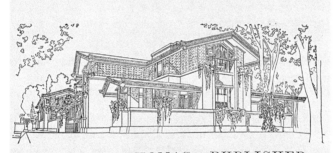

CHARLES C THOMAS · PUBLISHER
Springfield · Illinois · U.S.A.

FIG. 5.2 Title page of *Posttraumatic Epilepsy* (1949). *(Reproduced with permission from Walker AE, Posttraumatic epilepsy. Springfield, IL: Charles C. Thomas; 1949.)*

War II veterans with PTE. Next, Walker considers what is known about the risk factors for the development of PTE. Even at that time, it was clear that wounds penetrating the dura mater were associated with a much higher incidence of PTE than nonpenetrating injuries [6] (Chapter 2).

Walker next considers the neuropathology of the cicatrix. He indicates that:

As the result of a penetrating wound of the head…a firm scar forms between the dura mater and underlying brain. In many cases, a layer of blood in the subdural space becomes organized, forming a membrane of varying thickness. At the time of operation for a posttraumatic epilepsy, this subdural membrane is found firmly adherent to the dura mater. It may be 2–10mm in thickness and quite extensive overlying as much as one-half of a hemisphere in some cases or it may be of filamentous thinness (Fig. 5.3A). The brain adjoining the meningocerebral scar

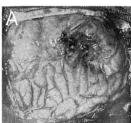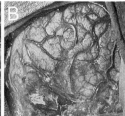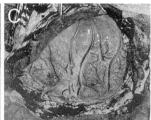

FIG. 5.3 Photographs of cortical scars reported by Walker in 1949. (A) Photograph of the exposed cerebral cortex to show a subdural membrane extending from the midline over the cortex, adjacent to a meningocerebral scar. (B) Photograph of the operative field showing areas of cerebral softening and arachnoidal calcification adjacent to an extensive scar. (C) Photograph of the exposed cortex, showing the severe arachnoidal proliferation adjoining a meningocortical scar. A subdural membrane has been reflected and covers the dura mater in the upper part of the illustration. *(Reproduced with permission from Walker AE. Posttraumatic epilepsy, Springfield, IL: Charles C. Thomas; 1949.)*

in some cases appears normal, but frequently it is yellow or brown, softened and
cystic (Fig. 5.3B). The arachnoid is often thickened and opaque, occasionally con-
taining white calcified plaques (Fig. 5.3C) [6].

Walker then explicitly references and endorses the mechanism described by Penfield and Foerster:

The scar in the cerebrum may be superficial or deep, but practically always it is
densely adherent to the overlying dura mater. As it contracts, this meningocer-
ebral cicatrix tugs on the adjacent brain. Foerster has demonstrated dilatation
and distortion at the site of the lesion, and the "wandering" of the entire ventricu-
lar system toward the cerebral scar. The mechanisms involved in the cicatricial
contraction of the brain have been clearly described by Wilder Penfield. The gross
alterations produced by a brain injury—the amount of brain substance lost, the
degree of ventricular distortion, and the state of the subarachnoid spaces—may be
demonstrated in man by pneumoencephalography [6].

Walker next reports the findings in the series of 246 posttraumatic epileptic patients studied at Cushing General Hospital. Of these, 109 had pneumoencephalograms taken. Overall, the most common pneumoencephalographic finding in cases of penetrating head injury was a bilateral ventricular enlargement with an outpouching at the site of the skull defect. However, Walker notes that the same findings could be observed in patients with TBI that had not developed PTE [14].

What about histological findings? Here, Walker states the following:

Histologically, the scar following a penetrating wound of the brain is composed of
a network of connective tissue, blood vessels and islands of glial tissue. Neurones
are rarely present. At the margin of the scar, the connective tissue elements become
less and are seen penetrating the glial scar which extends peripherally. At the

border of the scar the cerebral cortex appears grossly normal except for possibly arachnoidal thickening. When examined microscopically, this cortex is always abnormal. It consists of a decreased and degenerated neuronal complement with hyperplastic and hypertrophic astrocytes and gitter cells which Penfield considers evidence of progressive destruction. The epileptogenic zone in one sector of the margin of the scar cannot be distinguished histologically from the remainder of the marginal cortex [6].

This observation—that the epileptogenic zone could not be distinguished from the overall pathological changes in the brain as a response to the traumatic brain injury itself—led Walker to conclude that "it seems likely that the anatomical substrata of the epileptogenic focus are too subtle for demonstration by our present techniques" [6]. It does not escape attention, however, that the histology reported by Walker in 1949 (Fig. 5.4) appears no better and perhaps somewhat inferior to that reported by Foerster and Penfield 19 years earlier (Figs. 3.16 and 3.17) [1].

At the most experienced practitioner of his era, what was Walker's approach to the treatment of PTE? First, he emphasized that "the treatment of posttraumatic epilepsy is primarily medical" in other words with drug therapy. At the time (1949) the most common drugs used were phenobarbital and phenytoin [6]. Walker held that surgery was indicated in cases of "repair of skull defects

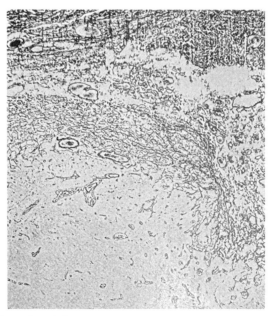

FIG. 5.4 Histology of cortical scar reported by Walker in 1949. Photomicrograph of the cortex adjacent to a scar, showing invasion of the cortex by reticular tissue. The arachnoid is markedly thickened over this area. Perdrau preparation, 55× magnification. *(Reproduced with permission from Walker AE. Posttraumatic epilepsy. Springfield, IL: Charles C. Thomas; 1949.)*

associated with the injury, the removal of foreign bodies, and the removal of cerebral scars or epileptogenic foci after medical therapy has failed to control the epilepsy" [6]. In the latter case, what was his surgical approach to cortical operations for PTE? Based on early electroencephalography (EEG) studies, Walker stated (*contra* the original conception of Foerster and Penfield) that

> *It is now recognized that the cortex, at the margin of the scar, is the source of the epileptic discharges in the electroencephalogram, and it is the area which, when stimulated, gives rise to the attack. This epileptogenic zone, not the scar, is the focus responsible for the epilepsy [6].*

This key distinction from Foerster and Penfield's hypothesis that "cicatricial contraction" or traction from the scar itself was responsible for the epilepsy led Walker to propose extirpation specifically of this epileptogenic zone. Walker admitted, however, that "the factors which cause one area of marginal cortex about a scar to become epileptogenic are unknown" [6].

Because of the necessity of identifying which areas of the adjacent cortex comprise the epileptogenic zone, Walker combined awake craniotomies with extensive intraoperative electrocorticography. He placed electrodes to sample both spontaneous and electrically induced activity in the perilesional cortex (Fig. 5.5). Spontaneous epileptiform spiking activity would demonstrate the presence of perilesional foci (Fig. 5.6).

Occasionally, stimulation of the perilesional foci would induce the patient's typical aura (and all of these patients were operated on awake to constantly assess symptoms and motor and speech functions). Once the epileptic focus had thus been located and its extent determined, Walker used one of three techniques: (1) excision of the focus and the scar to the ventricle (Fig. 5.7); (2) removal of the focus and the scar to normal white matter (Fig. 5.8); or (3) subpial resection of the focus (Figs. 5.9 and 5.10). The blood supply to the remaining cerebral cortex was disrupted as little as possible.

Using these electrocorticography-guided resections, Walker reported the following results in his 1949 monograph [6]. Of the 36 patients with medically-intractable PTE treated surgically, one-third (12/36) had no further seizures at 1 year postoperatively and another one-fifth (7/36) had only one seizure or just the aura of their seizure. Thus, 19 of 36 (53%) had what could be considered a good to excellent result from surgery. He compared a control group of 20 similar medically-intractable PTE patients treated without surgery, and only 3 of 20 (15%) had one or fewer attacks over the same interval [6]. These results compared favorably to another contemporary series of 26 cases of PTE treated surgically by Penfield and Steelman between 1939 and 1944 in which 50% (13/26) were either cured or markedly improved by cortical excisions [15]. Walker was careful to note that despite reporting the largest surgical series to date, "the ultimate value of the surgical treatment of posttraumatic epilepsy can only be determined after a five or ten year follow-up" [6].

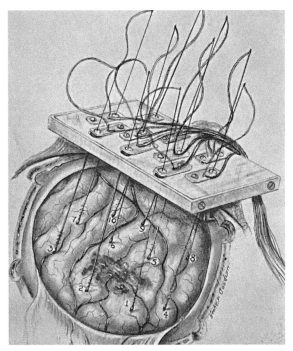

FIG. 5.5 The electrode holder is clamped to the margin of the calvarium and the electrodes placed upon the cortex for recording. *(Reproduced with permission from Walker AE. Posttraumatic epilepsy. Springfield, IL: Charles C. Thomas; 1949.)*

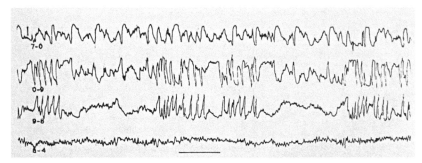

FIG. 5.6 Spontaneous electrocorticograms from an epileptogenous focus in the right inferior frontal region. The record shows out-of-phase spiking in the first three leads indicating two foci, one at point 0 and one at point 9. Such epileptic activity was infrequently found in the routine electrocorticograms. The horizontal line at the base indicates a second interval; the vertical line in the upper left-hand corner is a calibration of 50 microvolts. *(Reproduced with permission from Walker AE. Posttraumatic epilepsy. Springfield, IL: Charles C. Thomas; 1949.)*

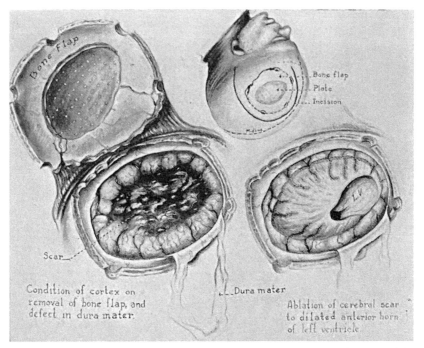

FIG. 5.7 Sketch of the operative field showing an extensive left frontal cerebral scar containing bone fragments. The scar was removed to the ventricle. *(Reproduced with permission from Walker AE. Posttraumatic epilepsy. Springfield, IL: Charles C. Thomas; 1949.)*

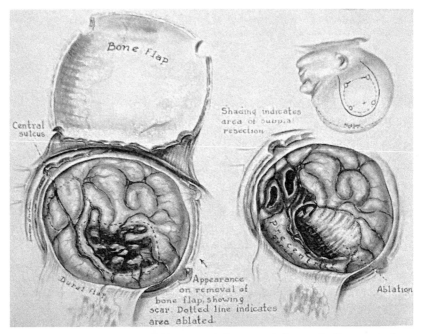

FIG. 5.8 Sketch of the operative field before and after removal of scar and epileptogenous focus. The wound was a bullet "crease" of the parietal bone without fracture of the bone. Despite the absence of penetration, a large scar was present in the parietal region. *(Reproduced with permission from Walker AE. Posttraumatic epilepsy. Springfield, IL: Charles C. Thomas; 1949.)*

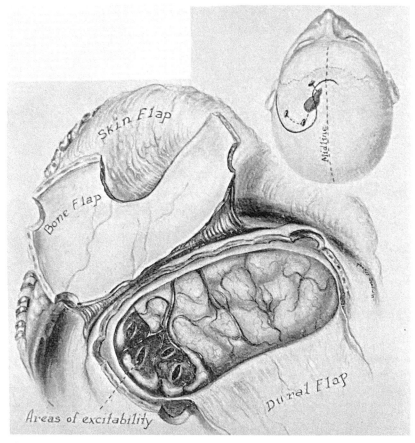

FIG. 5.9 Sketch to illustrate subpial resection of an epileptogenic focus adjacent to a scar. *(Reproduced with permission from Walker AE. Posttraumatic epilepsy. Springfield, IL: Charles C. Thomas; 1949.)*

Modern series of surgical treatments of posttraumatic epilepsy

Following the monumental contributions of Penfield and Walker, for several decades there were no significant publications specifically addressing the surgical treatment of PTE. In the following section, we summarize the modern series of PTE surgery and outcomes.

In 1995, the Yale epilepsy group reported on 25 patients who developed intractable complex partial seizures after head trauma. All patients underwent magnetic resonance imaging (MRI), neuropsychological evaluation, and surface EEG monitoring, and 21 of 25 also underwent intracranial EEG monitoring. Seizures were successfully localized in nine patients, all of whom underwent a surgical procedure and became seizure-free; six of nine had a mesial temporal lobe seizure focus, and three of nine had neocortical foci with circumscribed

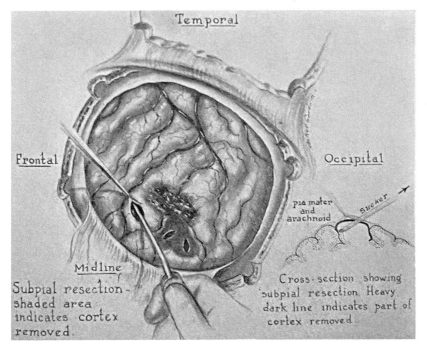

FIG. 5.10 The technique of subpial resection is illustrated. The cortical ablation is carried to the depth of the sulcus. *(Reproduced with permission from Walker AE. Posttraumatic epilepsy. Springfield, IL: Charles C. Thomas; 1949.)*

radiographic abnormalities. The remaining 16 patients did not have a focal MRI lesion and the seizures were not adequately localized. This study indicates that surgical outcomes using modern MRI and EEG can be excellent in the group of patients who have successful EEG localization of seizure onset and focal MRI findings [16].

In 1996, investigators from the Montreal Neurological Institute reported on six patients with large posttraumatic frontal lesions and intractable frontal lobe epilepsy (FLE) [17]. This group had intractable FLE related to direct impact head trauma and were selected based on abnormal imaging findings. In all six patients, neuroradiological studies showed focal atrophy, and in five of six frontal wedge-shaped gliotic lesions were present. Contralateral lesions were not observed on computerized tomography (CT) or MRI. EEG and intraoperative electrocorticography (ECoG) was used. Surgery consisted of removal of the visible scar and of surrounding gliotic tissue with additional ECoG guidance. The mean follow-up was 2.6 years (range 1–5 years). Five patients were seizure-free postoperatively, and the sixth had an 85% reduction in seizure frequency. No increase in frontal lobe deficits occurred as a result of surgery. The authors emphasized that the excellent results obtained in this series are likely the result of the focality of the lesions encountered and treated [17].

In 1997, a group of investigators reported a series of 17 consecutive patients who underwent resection of frontal encephalomalacias at Mayo Clinic-Rochester between 1987 and 1994 as treatment of intractable FLE [18]. All 17 patients underwent comprehensive presurgical evaluation including EEG, MRI, and intraoperative ECoG. The operative strategy was complete resection of the encephalomalacia together with the adjacent electrophysiologically abnormal tissues identified by interictal and ictal EEG and intraoperative ECoG. At a median of 3 years of follow-up (range 0.6–7.5 years), 12 patients (70%) were seizure-free or only had rare seizures. The authors concluded that surgery is very effective for intractable FLE secondary to encephalomalacias [18].

In 2008, Hartzfeld et al. retrospectively reviewed all patients with posttraumatic medial temporal lobe epilepsy (MTLE) operated for PTE over a 10-year period (1993–2003) within the Henry Ford Health System [19]. They found 57 patients who underwent surgery. Of the 57, 30 underwent medial temporal lobe resection. The most common mechanism of injury was blunt trauma attributable to motor vehicle accidents. Imaging abnormalities included mesial temporal sclerosis (MTS; 16 cases), T2/FLAIR (fluid-attenuated inversion recovery) hyperintensities (9 cases), periventricular gliosis (7 cases), diffuse cerebral atrophy (5 cases), and focal encephalomalacia (3 cases). Six patients had normal MRIs. No significant difference was found between the posttraumatic and nontraumatic MTLE surgery groups in the rate of freedom from disabling seizures postoperatively (64% vs 78%, respectively) [19].

In 2012, a retrospective study was done by the University of Washington epilepsy group of all epilepsy surgeries performed over a 17-year span that were associated with trauma or brain injury [20]. Inclusion criteria were adult patients who underwent extratemporal resection (with or without temporal lobectomy) in whom no other cause of epilepsy other than trauma could be identified. Twenty-one patients met inclusion and exclusion criteria. Six of 21 patients (28%) were seizure-free and 6 of 21 (28%) had a good outcome of two or fewer seizures per year. Another five patients (24%) experienced a reduction in seizures and four (19%) did not attain benefit. In the subset of eight patients with the combination of encephalomalacia and invasive intracranial EEG, five (62.5%) became seizure-free postoperatively. The authors concluded that many patients with extratemporal PTE can achieve good to excellent seizure control with epilepsy surgery, particularly those with focal encephalomalacia on MRI and resection guided by intracranial EEG to define the extent of resection [20].

In 2020, investigators from the University of Pennsylvania published a surgical PTE series [21]. This was a retrospective study of patients with a history of head injury undergoing surgical treatment for epilepsy. Twenty-three patients met the inclusion criteria. Nineteen (82.6%) had mesial temporal sclerosis, three (13.0%) had lesional neocortical epilepsy, and one (4.3%) had nonlesional cortical epilepsy; 14/23 (60.9%) underwent temporal lobectomy, two (8.7%) underwent cortical resection, and seven (30.4%) underwent vagus nerve stimulator

(VNS) implantation. Three patients subsequently underwent responsive neuro-stimulator (RNS) implantation after VNS failed to reduce seizure frequency by more than 50%. In patients treated with temporal lobectomy or cortical resection, 68.8% became seizure-free [21].

The largest modern series of resective surgery for drug-resistant PTE was published in 2020 by a group from Beijing [22]. The authors retrospectively reviewed the records of all patients with drug-resistant PTE who had undergone resective surgery at their institution between January 2008 and December 2016. Inclusion criteria were: (1) clear history of TBI preceding initial seizure onset; (2) evidence of trauma on preoperative imaging; and (3) patients who underwent resective surgery for drug-resistant PTE. All patients had at least a 2-year follow-up (mean follow-up 5.79 years, range 2–10 years). Of the 90 patients identified in this group, 63/90 (70%) were seizure-free over the follow-up period.

The above clinical studies and the available literature indicate that there are particular anatomic subtypes of medically-intractable PTE. These have been characterized as independent "neuroimaging endophenotypes" of PTE [23]. First, PTE may be associated with isolated temporal lobe epilepsy (TLE) with MTS with no other structural abnormalities (Fig. 5.11A). Second, there may be "dual pathology" with MTS found in addition to neocortical lesions, usually in temporal or frontal lobes (Fig. 5.11B and C). Third, there may be isolated extratemporal neocortical epilepsy (Fig. 5.12).

Case example: Surgical treatment of posttraumatic epilepsy

One of the authors of this book (D.K.B.) is a surgical epilepsy fellowship-trained neurosurgeon who has treated several cases of PTE with surgical resection. As described in the Kazemi *et al.* 1997 publication on successful resection

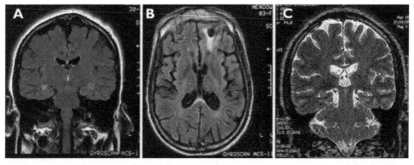

FIG. 5.11 Magnetic resonance imaging (MRI) findings in patients evaluated for intractable post-traumatic epilepsy. (A) Right hippocampal sclerosis and global cerebral atrophy. (B and C) (same patient) Coexistence of left frontal contusion and hemosiderosis with left hippocampal sclerosis. *(Reproduced with permission from Diaz-Arrastia R, et al. Posttraumatic epilepsy: the endophenotypes of a human model of epileptogenesis. Epilepsia 2009;50 Suppl 2:14–20.)*

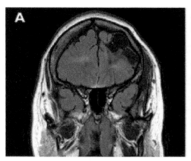 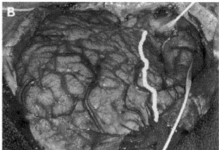

FIG. 5.12 Magnetic resonance imaging (MRI) and operative findings in a patient with posttraumatic epilepsy resulting from left frontal contusion. The patient was a 23-year-old woman who developed epilepsy at age 18 after a severe traumatic brain injury (TBI) in infancy that produced coma for 3 months. (A) MRI shows extensive left frontal encephalomalacia, as well as some global atrophy. (B) Intracranial monitoring with subdural electrodes localized zone of seizure onset and cortical mapping allowed localization of language and motor regions. Tailored cortical resection *(yellow line)* resulted in complete seizure control. *(Reproduced with permission from Diaz-Arrastia R, et al. Posttraumatic epilepsy: the endophenotypes of a human model of epileptogenesis. Epilepsia 2009;50 Suppl 2:14–20.)*

of frontal encephalomalacias [18], in cases of epileptogenic frontal lobe damage surgical resection may be curative. One such case can serve to illustrate this point and the potential for excellent outcomes in this PTE patient subgroup.

A 44-year-old man presented with medically-intractable epilepsy. He had a severe TBI with a closed head injury at age 16 from a bicycle accident associated with a prolonged loss of consciousness (3 days). He started to have recurrent stereotyped seizures at age 19. The seizures began with an aura consisting of an unpleasant "chemical" taste and smell, fear, and binaural auditory distortion followed by impairment of consciousness associated with behavioral arrest, unresponsiveness, and postictal confusion. At presentation, these complex partial seizures were occurring 4–6 times per week, and secondary generalization with tonic-clonic seizures occurred at least once per month.

Imaging demonstrated cystic encephalomalacia in the right frontal lobe (Fig. 5.13). This included a dark rim on T2-weighted imaging consistent with hemosiderin, suggesting that this was an epileptogenic cyst from an old frontal contusion (Fig. 5.14). Interestingly, imaging also demonstrated right mesial temporal sclerosis (Fig. 5.15), indicating "dual pathology". Phase 2 monitoring was performed with extensive coverage of the right frontal lobe, left frontal lobe, and bilateral mesial temporal regions to identify the seizure onset zone (Fig. 5.16).

Several typical seizures were recorded during Phase 2 video-EEG monitoring in the epilepsy monitoring unit. This revealed typical seizure onset around the right frontal cyst *without* independent seizure onset in the temporal lobe. Therefore, the surgical decision was made to limit resection to complete removal of the epileptogenic cyst and *not* to perform mesial temporal resection

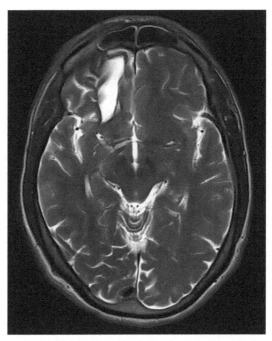

FIG. 5.13 Preoperative axial T2-weighted image demonstrates right frontal cystic encephalomalacia.

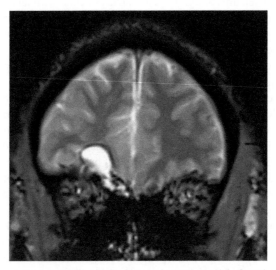

FIG. 5.14 Preoperative coronal T2-weighted image demonstrates right frontal cyst with dark hemosiderin rim.

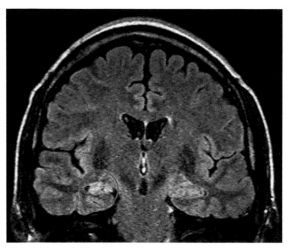

FIG. 5.15 Preoperative coronal FLAIR image demonstrates right mesial temporal sclerosis *(red circle)*.

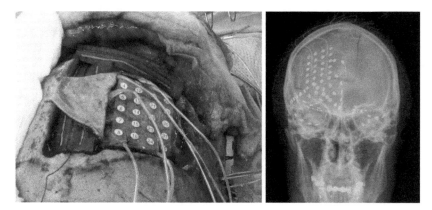

FIG. 5.16 Craniotomy for electrode placement (Phase 2 monitoring) was performed including placement of right frontal grid and strip electrodes and right temporal depth electrodes *(left, in-traoperative photograph)* and left frontal strips and left temporal depth electrodes as well *(right, postoperative anteroposterior skull X-ray showing extensive bilateral electrode coverage)*.

in this case. A second craniotomy was performed for the removal of electrodes and cyst resection. Following the removal of the electrodes, pial incision was made in the right frontal lobe over the cyst (Fig. 5.17A). The cyst was accessed and found to be surrounded by a yellow hemosiderin rim (Fig. 5.17B and C). Resection of the entire cyst and hemosiderin rim was performed (Fig. 5.17D).

Postoperative imaging demonstrated resection confined to the epileptogenic right frontal cyst (Fig. 5.18). The patient was discharged from the hospital on postresection day #2. He had no neuropsychological deficits. Since the procedure, he has only had two auras (simple partial seizures) but no complex partial

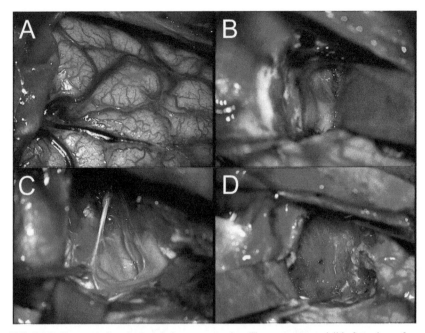

FIG. 5.17 Intraoperative pictures during cyst resection. The cyst was not visible from the surface of the right frontal lobe (A), but following corticectomy the cyst was found deep to the cortex (B). Yellow hemosiderin staining was seen around the wall of the cyst (B, C) and complete removal of the cyst and surrounding hemosiderin-stained rim was performed (D).

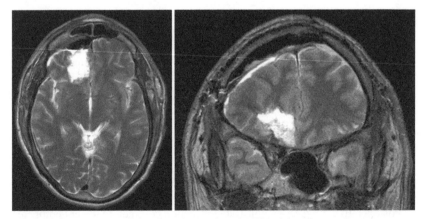

FIG. 5.18 Postoperative axial (*left*) and coronal (*right*) T2-weighted images demonstrate complete removal of the right frontal epileptogenic cyst.

seizures (with loss of consciousness) and no generalized tonic-clonic seizures. Thus, he is free of disabling seizures postoperatively. His quality of life has significantly improved.

Perspective

Overall, PTE can be categorized into temporal lobe epilepsy and nontemporal lobe epilepsy, and separately into lesional and nonlesional, with MTS as a specific lesional category within TLE [21,23]. Available studies indicate that TLE is the most commonly reported subtype in a series of PTE, and MTS is observed in approximately half of these patients [21,23,24]. Surgical treatment of TLE with or without a history of prior head trauma is associated with good to excellent outcomes [19,25,26]. It is also clear, however, that nontemporal PTE may also be amenable to surgical treatment. In particular, the series on frontal lobe lesions and encephalomalacias causing FLE as a subtype of PTE demonstrate excellent outcomes following focal lesional frontal lobe resection guided by EEG [17,18]. It is apparent that "surgery may currently be underutilized as treatment of severely disabling epilepsy in patients with frontal encephalomalacias" [18]. Whatever the location of onset (temporal or nontemporal), the best surgical outcomes in PTE surgery involve focal lesions on MRI and resection carefully tailored by preoperative and intraoperative electrophysiology [27]. Thus, despite the heterogeneity of TBI and PTE, modern epilepsy surgery utilizing state-of-the-art imaging and electrophysiology can be successfully employed in cases of PTE amenable to tailored surgical resection. Given the epidemiology of PTE in military and civilian populations (Chapter 2) and its intractable nature in many cases, it is difficult to escape the conclusion that surgery for PTE is underutilized.

References

[1] Foerster O, Penfield W. The structural basis of traumatic epilepsy and results of radical operation. Brain 1930;53:99–119.

[2] Walker AE. The primate thalamus. Chicago, IL: University of Chicago Press; 1938.

[3] Walker AE, Taggart JK. Congenital atresia of the foramens of Luschka and Magendie. Arch Neurol Psychiatry 1942;48:583–612.

[4] Walker AE. Lissencephaly. Arch Neurol Psychiatry 1942;48:13–29.

[5] Walker AE, et al. Convulsive effects of antibiotic agents on the cerebral cortex. Science 1946;103:116.

[6] Walker AE. Posttraumatic epilepsy. Springfield, IL: Charles C. Thomas; 1949.

[7] Walker AE, editor. A history of neurological surgery. Baltimore, MD: The Williams & Wilkins Company; 1951.

[8] Black P, Shepard R, Walker AE. Outcome of head trauma: age and posttraumatic seizures. In: Porter R, Fitzsimon DW, editors. Outcome of severe damage to the central nervous system. Amsterdam: Elsevier; 1975. p. 215–26.

[9] Caveness WF, Walker AE, Ascroft PB. Incidence of posttraumatic epilepsy in Korean veterans as compared with those from World War I and World War II. J Neurosurg 1962;19:122–9.

[10] Feeney DM, Walker AE. The prediction of posttraumatic epilepsy. A mathematical approach. Arch Neurol 1979;36(1):8–12.

[11] Walker AE. Posttraumatic epilepsy in World War II veterans. Surg Neurol 1989;32(3):235–6.

[12] Walker AE, Jablon S. A follow-up of head injured men of World War II. J Neurosurg 1959;16:600–10.

[13] Walker AE, Jablon S. Follow-up study of head wounds in World War II. Washington, DC: The National Academies Press; 1961.

[14] Troland CE, Baxter DH, Schatzki R. Observations on encephalographic findings in cerebral trauma. J Neurosurg 1946;3:390–8.

[15] Penfield W, Steelman H. The treatment of focal epilepsy by cortical excision. Ann Surg 1947;126:740–62.

[16] Marks DA, et al. Seizure localization and pathology following head injury in patients with uncontrolled epilepsy. Neurology 1995;45(11):2051–7.

[17] Cukiert A, Olivier A, Andermann F. Post-traumatic frontal lobe epilepsy with structural changes: excellent results after cortical resection. Can J Neurol Sci 1996;23(2):114–7.

[18] Kazemi NJ, et al. Resection of frontal encephalomalacias for intractable epilepsy: outcome and prognostic factors. Epilepsia 1997;38(6):670–7.

[19] Hartzfeld P, et al. Characteristics and surgical outcomes for medial temporal post-traumatic epilepsy. Br J Neurosurg 2008;22(2):224–30.

[20] Hakimian S, et al. Long-term outcome of extratemporal resection in posttraumatic epilepsy. Neurosurg Focus 2012;32(3):E10.

[21] Hitti FL, et al. Surgical outcomes in post-traumatic epilepsy: a single institutional experience. Oper Neurosurg (Hagerstown) 2020;18(1):12–8.

[22] He X, et al. Resective surgery for drug-resistant posttraumatic epilepsy: predictors of seizure outcome. J Neurosurg 2019;1–8.

[23] Diaz-Arrastia R, et al. Posttraumatic epilepsy: the endophenotypes of a human model of epileptogenesis. Epilepsia 2009;50(Suppl 2):14–20.

[24] Diaz-Arrastia R, et al. Neurophysiologic and neuroradiologic features of intractable epilepsy after traumatic brain injury in adults. Arch Neurol 2000;57(11):1611–6.

[25] Engel Jr J, et al. Early surgical therapy for drug-resistant temporal lobe epilepsy: a randomized trial. JAMA 2012;307(9):922–30.

[26] Wiebe S, et al. A randomized, controlled trial of surgery for temporal-lobe epilepsy. N Engl J Med 2001;345(5):311–8.

[27] Rao VR, Parko KL. Clinical approach to posttraumatic epilepsy. Semin Neurol 2015;35(1):57–63.

Chapter 6

Animal models of traumatic brain injury

Overview

Posttraumatic epilepsy (PTE) is a long-term negative consequence of traumatic brain injury (TBI) in which recurrent spontaneous seizures occur after the initial head injury. Animal models have been used to study TBI for over a century [1–4] and provide a unique opportunity for researchers to investigate the pathophysiological changes by which trauma leads to PTE. Although preclinical models cannot entirely recapitulate the human condition, they are essential for understanding the biomechanical, cellular, and molecular mechanisms underlying TBI and the development of PTE. In this chapter, we will review the six most widely used mechanical TBI animal models: fluid percussion injury, controlled cortical impact injury, weight drop injury, penetrating ballistic-like injury, blast-induced injury, and undercut injury.

Fluid percussion injury

Fluid percussion injury (FPI) is one of the oldest models of TBI. FPI is generally used to replicate human closed head injury, producing both focal and diffuse (mixed) brain injury. Historically, FPI was developed for use in cats [5–7] and then adapted for use in dogs [8,9], sheep [9], swine [10], rabbits [11–13], rats [14–16], and mice [17]. The FPI model (Fig. 6.1) uses a pendulum, dropped from a predetermined height, to strike the piston of a cylindrical fluid reservoir that generates a fluid pressure pulse onto the intact dura [18]. The degree of the injury is dependent on the strength of the pressure pulse allowing for a reproducible injury [19–22].

Controlled cortical impact injury

The controlled cortical impact (CCI) injury model replicates a focal open or closed head injury, in which the damage is caused by a mechanically driven piston [23,24]. The model was first developed for use in ferrets [25], then expanded to mice [26,27], rats [28], swine [29], and nonhuman primates [30]. In this model, the injury is delivered to the intact dura using a pneumatic or electromagnetically driven actuator to induce a well-controlled injury [31,32]

Posttraumatic Epilepsy. https://doi.org/10.1016/B978-0-323-90099-7.00009-5

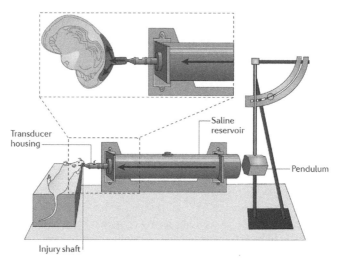

FIG. 6.1 Experimental set-up for fluid percussion injury. *(Reproduced with permission from Xiong YA, et al. Animal models of traumatic brain injury. Nat Rev Neurosci 2013;14(2):128–142.)*

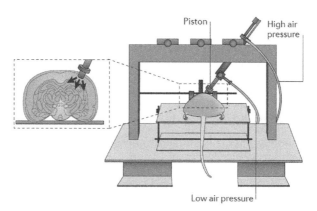

FIG. 6.2 Experimental set-up for controlled cortical impact injury. *(Reproduced with permission from Xiong YA, et al. Animal models of traumatic brain injury. Nat Rev Neurosci 2013;14(2):128–42.)*

(Fig. 6.2). The CCI model is used widely due to its high reproducibility, relative ease of use, and high survivability after injury induction [33]. It allows the user to adjust mechanical factors such as velocity of impact, depth of impact, diameter of the impactor tip, and duration of contact, which results in a reproducible level of injury [34].

Weight drop injury

The weight drop injury (WDI) model has been developed to replicate the impact acceleration/deceleration force of the brain to generate a focal or diffuse injury in rodents [35,36] and most recently has been modified for use in zebrafish [37,38]. The WDI model utilizes a guided free-falling weight from a designated height in which the degree of injury is determined by the mass of the weight and the height at which it is released [39]. Several variations of the WDI model include Feeney's, Shohami's, and Marmarou's weight drop models.

Feeney model

The Feeney WDI model (Fig. 6.3) was the first to be developed and involves a focal injury to the intact dura, resulting in a cortical contusion [40]. In Feeney's weight drop model, the weight strikes a footplate positioned over the exposed dura generating cortical cavitation after injury [41].

Shohami model

The Shohami WDI model uses a focal closed head injury in which a blunt injury is induced on one side of the unprotected skull while the head of the animal is placed on a hard surface during the impact [42,43].

Marmarou model

The Marmarou WDI model (Fig. 6.4) represents a closed head acceleration injury that results in diffuse axonal injury. In this model, a metal disk helmet is affixed to the skull, and the head of the animal is placed on a flexible platform to allow for rotational acceleration [44,45].

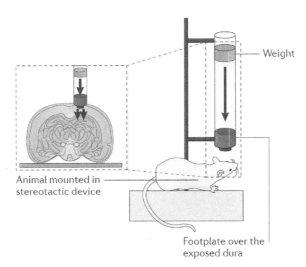

FIG. 6.3 Experimental set-up for Feeney weight drop injury. *(Reproduced with permission from Xiong YA, et al. Animal models of traumatic brain injury. Nat Rev Neurosci 2013;14(2):128–42.)*

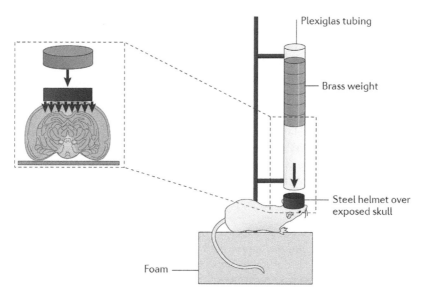

FIG. 6.4 Experimental set-up for Marmarou weight drop injury. *(Reproduced with permission from Xiong YA, et al. Animal models of traumatic brain injury. Nat Rev Neurosci 2013;14(2):128–42.)*

Penetrating ballistic-like brain injury

Penetrating ballistic-like brain injury (PBBI) is a focal open or closed head injury in which the damage is caused by the overpressure from penetrating low- or high-velocity projectiles [46]. PBBI models have been established to study the mechanisms of ballistic shock wave impact and/or the effect of a projectile penetrating the brain. A wide range of animal species have been utilized for PBBI research including mice [47], rats [48,49], cats [46,50], dogs [51], sheep [52,53], swine [54], and nonhuman primates [55,56].

Ballistic shock wave

The ballistic shock wave PBBI model (Fig. 6.5) simulates the temporary cavity caused by the kinetics of a ballistic shock wave [57]. This injury is induced in animals through a balloon tip probe inserted in a cranial window at the desired location, at which a silastic balloon is inflated and deflated rapidly [58–63].

Projectiles

The projectile PBBI model has also been established to study the permanent injury tract created by a projectile. Historically, bullets were used for large animal studies due to their size. Studies involving rodents have employed several methods to mimic stab wounds created by a dissecting knife [64], scalpel blade [65], needle [66], and wire knife [67]. Some studies induce injury with a copper wire drilled into the skull [68], while others employ a modified air rifle to project a pellet into the brain [69] (Fig. 6.6). Altogether, these study methods produce heterogeneous injuries making it difficult to fully understand the mechanism for each type of penetrating injury.

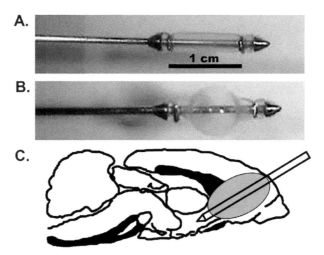

FIG. 6.5   Experimental set-up for penetrating ballistic-like brain injury (PBBI) model using a balloon tip probe. (A) PBBI probe. (B) PBBI probe with balloon inflation. (C) Anatomical location of injury tract with probe alone and probe with balloon inflation. *(Reproduced with permission from Cartagena CM, et al. Subacute changes in cleavage processing of amyloid precursor protein and tau following penetrating traumatic brain injury. PLoS One 2016;11(7):e0158576.)*

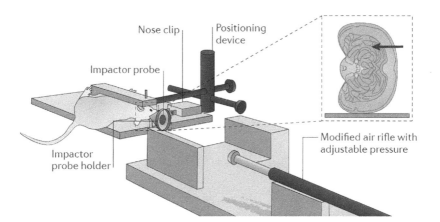

FIG. 6.6   Experimental set-up for penetrating ballistic-like brain injury using a projectile. *(Reproduced with permission from Xiong YA, et al. Animal models of traumatic brain injury. Nat Rev Neurosci 2013;14(2):128–42.)*

Blast-induced traumatic brain injury

Primary blast-induced traumatic brain injury (bTBI) is a diffuse closed head injury in which the damage is a direct effect of changes in overpressure caused by a blast wave [70]. Blast TBI is separate and distinct from other forms of TBI. Explosions are dynamic and may affect other body regions, making bTBI the most challenging model to reproduce and recapitulate the human condition [71–73]. A wide range of animal species have been utilized for bTBI research including mice [74,75], rats [76], ferrets [77], rabbits [78], swine [79,80], sheep [81], goats [82], and nonhuman primates [83]. Primary blast injury can be induced in animals through field explosives to simulate battlefield conditions [84–86] or shock tubes to approximate blast conditions [87].

Shock tubes

The shock tube induction system (Fig. 6.7) routinely used in the blast exposure model consists of a cylindrical metal tube in which animals are fixed into position to prevent rotational acceleration forces and exposed to the propagation of blast-like wave pressure driven by compressed air, gas, or explosive charges [88–91]. The shock tube paradigm and species used, location of the specimen, head mobility, body shielding, and overall complexity of generated waveforms may affect the nature of the injury creating variability among researchers [92–98]. This wide range of experimental variables limits reproducibility.

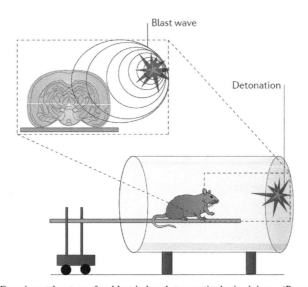

FIG. 6.7 Experimental set-up for blast-induced traumatic brain injury. *(Reproduced with permission from Xiong YA, et al. Animal models of traumatic brain injury. Nat Rev Neurosci 2013;14(2):128–42.)*

Undercut traumatic brain injury

The undercut traumatic brain injury model has been established to study cortical and white matter lesions. This method has been utilized in cats [99–103], guinea pigs [104], rats [105–110], and mice [111,112]. In this model, the damage is surgically induced by a transcortical incision in the sensorimotor cortex to create a lesion in the white matter or at the junction of the cortex. This injury results in partially isolated cortical regions (islands) from the surrounding cortex and subcortical regions [113] (Fig. 6.8).

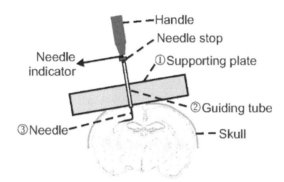

FIG. 6.8 Structure and application of an undercut device. A guiding tube (2) is glued onto a supporting plate (1) that is made of stainless steel or transparent plastic. A syringe needle (3) is inserted through the guiding tube (2) and bent at ~3 mm to the tip. A needle stop made of a plastic tube is glued onto the upper end of the needle so that the vertical moving range of the needle is limited to ~1.2 mm and ~1.5 mm for use in P21 mice and rats, respectively. A segment of small copper wire is fastened beneath the handle as a needle indicator for the orientation of the bent needle. Note that the device is tilted and in contact with both edges of the cranial window so that a cut can be made parallel to the pial surface. *(Reproduced with permission from Xiong W, et al. Preparing undercut model of posttraumatic epileptogenesis in rodents, J Vis Exp 2011;55.)*

Over the past few decades, animal models of TBI have been developed and modified, and novel models established to increase our understanding of dynamic processes underlying brain injury across species [114–116]. Most recently, a closed head injury model has been developed using pulsed high-intensity focused ultrasound (pHIFU) to induce TBI in zebrafish [117,118]. Another closed head injury model has been established using a piezoelectric actuator to deliver a compression force to the head of a fly [119]. These recent findings are promising; however, further study is needed to evaluate these models. To date, there is no single animal model which completely recapitulates the pathological, cellular, and molecular changes that occur in human TBI. Although heterogeneity in human TBI makes it difficult to model reproducibly, preclinical animal models are required to elucidate neurobiological mechanisms of TBI to improve our understanding of the development of PTE.

References

[1] Kramer SP. VI. A contribution to the theory of cerebral concussion. Ann Surg 1896;23(2):163–73.

[2] Denny-Brown DE, Russell WR. Experimental concussion: (section of neurology). Proc R Soc Med 1941;34(11):691–2.

[3] White JC, et al. Changes in brain volume and blood content after experimental concussion. Ann Surg 1943;118(4):619–33.

[4] Rinder L, Olsson Y. Studies on vascular permeability changes in experimental brain concussion. I. Distribution of circulating fluorescent indicators in brain and cervical cord after sudden mechanical loading of the brain. Acta Neuropathol 1968;11(3):183–200.

[5] Povlishock JT, Kontos HA. Continuing axonal and vascular change following experimental brain trauma. Cent Nerv Syst Trauma 1985;2(4):285–98.

[6] Hayes RL, et al. A new model of concussive brain injury in the cat produced by extradural fluid volume loading: II. Physiological and neuropathological observations. Brain Inj 1987;1(1):93–112.

[7] Sullivan HG, et al. Fluid-percussion model of mechanical brain injury in the cat. J Neurosurg 1976;45(5):521–34.

[8] Gurdjian ES, et al. Studies on experimental concussion: relation of physiologic effect to time duration of intracranial pressure increase at impact. Neurology 1954;4(9):674–81.

[9] Millen JE, Glauser FL, Fairman RP. A comparison of physiological responses to percussive brain trauma in dogs and sheep. J Neurosurg 1985;62(4):587–91.

[10] Pfenninger EG, et al. Early changes of intracranial pressure, perfusion pressure, and blood flow after acute head injury. Part 1: an experimental study of the underlying pathophysiology. J Neurosurg 1989;70(5):774–9.

[11] Lindgren S, Rinder L. Production and distribution of intracranial and intraspinal pressure changes at sudden extradural fluid volume input in rabbits. Acta Physiol Scand 1969;76(3):340–51.

[12] Stalhammar D. Experimental brain damage from fluid pressures due to impact acceleration. 1. Design of experimental procedure. Acta Neurol Scand 1975;52(1):7–26.

[13] Hartl R, et al. Early white blood cell dynamics after traumatic brain injury: effects on the cerebral microcirculation. J Cereb Blood Flow Metab 1997;17(11):1210–20.

[14] Dixon CE, et al. A fluid percussion model of experimental brain injury in the rat. J Neurosurg 1987;67(1):110–9.

[15] McIntosh TK, et al. Traumatic brain injury in the rat: characterization of a midline fluid-percussion model. Cent Nerv Syst Trauma 1987;4(2):119–34.

[16] Perri BR, et al. Metabolic quantification of lesion volume following experimental traumatic brain injury in the rat. J Neurotrauma 1997;14(1):15–22.

[17] Carbonell WS, et al. Adaptation of the fluid percussion injury model to the mouse. J Neurotrauma 1998;15(3):217–29.

[18] Kabadi SV, et al. Fluid-percussion-induced traumatic brain injury model in rats. Nat Protoc 2010;5(9):1552–63.

[19] McIntosh TK, et al. Traumatic brain injury in the rat: characterization of a lateral fluid-percussion model. Neuroscience 1989;28(1):233–44.

[20] Carbonell WS, Grady MS. Regional and temporal characterization of neuronal, glial, and axonal response after traumatic brain injury in the mouse. Acta Neuropathol 1999;98(4):396–406.

[21] Kharatishvili I, et al. A model of posttraumatic epilepsy induced by lateral fluid-percussion brain injury in rats. Neuroscience 2006;140(2):685–97.

[22] Alder J, et al. Lateral fluid percussion: model of traumatic brain injury in mice. J Vis Exp 2011;54.

[23] Chen Y, et al. A modified controlled cortical impact technique to model mild traumatic brain injury mechanics in mice. Front Neurol 2014;5:100.

[24] Szu JI, et al. Modulation of posttraumatic epileptogenesis in aquaporin-4 knockout mice. Epilepsia 2020;61(7):1503–14.

[25] Lighthall JW. Controlled cortical impact: a new experimental brain injury model. J Neurotrauma 1988;5(1):1–15.

[26] Smith DH, et al. A model of parasagittal controlled cortical impact in the mouse: cognitive and histopathologic effects. J Neurotrauma 1995;12(2):169–78.

[27] Hall ED, et al. Spatial and temporal characteristics of neurodegeneration after controlled cortical impact in mice: more than a focal brain injury. J Neurotrauma 2005;22(2):252–65.

[28] Dixon CE, et al. A controlled cortical impact model of traumatic brain injury in the rat. J Neurosci Methods 1991;39(3):253–62.

[29] Alessandri B, et al. Moderate controlled cortical contusion in pigs: effects on multiparametric neuromonitoring and clinical relevance. J Neurotrauma 2003;20(12):1293–305.

[30] King C, et al. Brain temperature profiles during epidural cooling with the ChillerPad in a monkey model of traumatic brain injury. J Neurotrauma 2010;27(10):1895–903.

[31] Szu JI, et al. Aquaporin-4 dysregulation in a controlled cortical impact injury model of posttraumatic epilepsy. Neuroscience 2020;428:140–53.

[32] Mohamed AZ, Cumming P, Nasrallah FA. Traumatic brain injury augurs ill for prolonged deficits in the brain's structural and functional integrity following controlled cortical impact injury. Sci Rep 2021;11(1):21559.

[33] Osier N, Dixon CE. The controlled cortical impact model of experimental brain trauma: overview, research applications, and protocol. Methods Mol Biol 2016;1462:177–92.

[34] Goodman JC, et al. Lateral cortical impact injury in rats: pathologic effects of varying cortical compression and impact velocity. J Neurotrauma 1994;11(5):587–97.

[35] Shapira Y, et al. Experimental closed head injury in rats: mechanical, pathophysiologic, and neurologic properties. Crit Care Med 1988;16(3):258–65.

[36] Foda MA, Marmarou A. A new model of diffuse brain injury in rats. Part II: morphological characterization. J Neurosurg 1994;80(2):301–13.

[37] Hentig J, et al. Zebrafish blunt-force TBI induces heterogenous injury pathologies that mimic human TBI and responds with sonic hedgehog-dependent cell proliferation across the neuroaxis. Biomedicine 2021;9(8).

[38] Hentig J, et al. A scalable model to study the effects of blunt-force injury in adult zebrafish. J Vis Exp 2021;171.

[39] Wang HC, et al. A new rat model for diffuse axonal injury using a combination of linear acceleration and angular acceleration. J Neurotrauma 2010;27(4):707–19.

[40] Feeney DM, et al. Responses to cortical injury: I. Methodology and local effects of contusions in the rat. Brain Res 1981;211(1):67–77.

[41] Xiong Y, Mahmood A, Chopp M. Animal models of traumatic brain injury. Nat Rev Neurosci 2013;14(2):128–42.

[42] Khalin I, et al. A mouse model of weight-drop closed head injury: emphasis on cognitive and neurological deficiency. Neural Regen Res 2016;11(4):630–5.

[43] Shohami E, Shapira Y, Cotev S. Experimental closed head injury in rats: prostaglandin production in a noninjured zone. Neurosurgery 1988;22(5):859–63.

[44] Piper IR, Thomson D, Miller JD. Monitoring weight drop velocity and foam stiffness as an aid to quality control of a rodent model of impact acceleration neurotrauma. J Neurosci Methods 1996;69(2):171–4.

[45] Hsieh TH, et al. Relationship of mechanical impact magnitude to neurologic dysfunction severity in a rat traumatic brain injury model. PLoS One 2017;12(5), e0178186.

[46] Carey ME, Sarna GS, Farrell JB. Brain edema following an experimental missile wound to the brain. J Neurotrauma 1990;7(1):13–20.

[47] Cernak I, et al. A novel mouse model of penetrating brain injury. Front Neurol 2014;5:209.

[48] Zoltewicz JS, et al. Biomarkers track damage after graded injury severity in a rat model of penetrating brain injury. J Neurotrauma 2013;30(13):1161–9.

[49] Cartagena CM, et al. Subacute changes in cleavage processing of amyloid precursor protein and tau following penetrating traumatic brain injury. PLoS One 2016;11(7), e0158576.

[50] Carey ME, et al. Experimental missile wound to the brain. J Neurosurg 1989;71(5 Pt 1):754–64.

[51] Tan Y, et al. A gross and microscopic study of cerebral injuries accompanying maxillofacial high-velocity projectile wounding in dogs. J Oral Maxillofac Surg 1998;56(3):345–8.

[52] Finnie JW. Pathology of experimental traumatic craniocerebral missile injury. J Comp Pathol 1993;108(1):93–101.

[53] Lazarjan MS, et al. Visualization of the air ejected from the temporary cavity in brain and tissue simulants during gunshot wounding. Forensic Sci Int 2015;246:104–9.

[54] Lu H, et al. Establishment of swine-penetrating craniocerebral gunshot wound model. J Surg Res 2015;199(2):698–706.

[55] Crockard HA, et al. An experimental cerebral missile injury model in primates. J Neurosurg 1977;46(6):776–83.

[56] Allen IV, Scott R, Tanner JA. Experimental high-velocity missile head injury. Injury 1982;14(2):183–93.

[57] Moshang E, Ling G, Groer J. A model of penetrating traumatic brain injury using an air inflation technique. Springfield, VA: National Technical Information Service; 2003. DAMD17-01-1-0742.

[58] Williams AJ, et al. Characterization of a new rat model of penetrating ballistic brain injury. J Neurotrauma 2005;22(2):313–31.

[59] Williams AJ, Ling GS, Tortella FC. Severity level and injury track determine outcome following a penetrating ballistic-like brain injury in the rat. Neurosci Lett 2006;408(3):183–8.

[60] Wei G, et al. Intracranial pressure following penetrating ballistic-like brain injury in rats. J Neurotrauma 2010;27(9):1635–41.

[61] Boutte AM, et al. Serum glial fibrillary acidic protein predicts tissue glial fibrillary acidic protein break-down products and therapeutic efficacy after penetrating ballistic-like brain injury. J Neurotrauma 2016;33(1):147–56.

[62] Spurlock MS, et al. Amelioration of penetrating ballistic-like brain injury induced cognitive deficits after neuronal differentiation of transplanted human neural stem cells. J Neurotrauma 2017;34(11):1981–95.

[63] Pandya JD, et al. Comprehensive profile of acute mitochondrial dysfunction in a preclinical model of severe penetrating TBI. Front Neurol 2019;10:605.

[64] Amat JA, et al. Phenotypic diversity and kinetics of proliferating microglia and astrocytes following cortical stab wounds. Glia 1996;16(4):368–82.

[65] Eugenin EA, et al. Microglia at brain stab wounds express connexin 43 and in vitro form functional gap junctions after treatment with interferon-gamma and tumor necrosis factor-alpha. Proc Natl Acad Sci U S A 2001;98(7):4190–5.

[66] Horvat A, et al. A novel role for protein tyrosine phosphatase shp1 in controlling glial activation in the normal and injured nervous system. J Neurosci 2001;21(3):865–74.

[67] Grossman R, et al. Persistent region-dependent neuroinflammation, NMDA receptor loss and atrophy in an animal model of penetrating brain injury. Future Neurol 2012;7(3):329–39.

[68] Kendirli MT, Rose DT, Bertram EH. A model of posttraumatic epilepsy after penetrating brain injuries: effect of lesion size and metal fragments. Epilepsia 2014;55(12):1969–77.

[69] Plantman S, et al. Characterization of a novel rat model of penetrating traumatic brain injury. J Neurotrauma 2012;29(6):1219–32.

[70] Celander H, et al. The use of a compressed air operated shock tube for physiological blast research. Acta Physiol Scand 1955;33(1):6–13.

[71] Svetlov SI, et al. Morphologic and biochemical characterization of brain injury in a model of controlled blast overpressure exposure. J Trauma 2010;69(4):795–804.

[72] Saljo A, et al. Mechanisms and pathophysiology of the low-level blast brain injury in animal models. Neuroimage 2011;54(Suppl 1):S83–8.

[73] Gullotti DM, et al. Significant head accelerations can influence immediate neurological impairments in a murine model of blast-induced traumatic brain injury. J Biomech Eng 2014;136(9), 091004.

[74] Hue CD, et al. Time course and size of blood-brain barrier opening in a mouse model of blast-induced traumatic brain injury. J Neurotrauma 2016;33(13):1202–11.

[75] Zhou Y, et al. Blast-induced traumatic brain injury triggered by moderate intensity shock wave using a modified experimental model of injury in mice. Chin Med J (Engl) 2018;131(20):2447–60.

[76] Kaur C, et al. Ultrastructural changes of macroglial cells in the rat brain following an exposure to a non-penetrative blast. Ann Acad Med Singapore 1997;26(1):27–9.

[77] Rafaels KA, et al. Brain injury risk from primary blast. J Trauma Acute Care Surg 2012;73(4):895–901.

[78] Cernak I. The importance of systemic response in the pathobiology of blast-induced neurotrauma. Front Neurol 2010;1:151.

[79] Bauman RA, et al. An introductory characterization of a combat-casualty-care relevant swine model of closed head injury resulting from exposure to explosive blast. J Neurotrauma 2009;26(6):841–60.

[80] de Lanerolle NC, et al. Characteristics of an explosive blast-induced brain injury in an experimental model. J Neuropathol Exp Neurol 2011;70(11):1046–57.

[81] Savic J, et al. Pathophysiologic reactions in sheep to blast waves from detonation of aerosol explosives. Vojnosanit Pregl 1991;48(6):499–506.

[82] Li BC, et al. Blast-induced traumatic brain injury of goats in confined space. Neurol Res 2014;36(11):974–82.

[83] Lu J, et al. Effect of blast exposure on the brain structure and cognition in *Macaca fascicularis*. J Neurotrauma 2012;29(7):1434–54.

[84] Kaur C, et al. The response of neurons and microglia to blast injury in the rat brain. Neuropathol Appl Neurobiol 1995;21(5):369–77.

[85] Cheng J, et al. Development of a rat model for studying blast-induced traumatic brain injury. J Neurol Sci 2010;294(1–2):23–8.

[86] Rubovitch V, et al. A mouse model of blast-induced mild traumatic brain injury. Exp Neurol 2011;232(2):280–9.

[87] Mishra V, et al. Primary blast causes mild, moderate, severe and lethal TBI with increasing blast overpressures: experimental rat injury model. Sci Rep 2016;6:26992.

[88] Garman RH, et al. Blast exposure in rats with body shielding is characterized primarily by diffuse axonal injury. J Neurotrauma 2011;28(6):947–59.

[89] Kuehn R, et al. Rodent model of direct cranial blast injury. J Neurotrauma 2011;28(10):2155–69.

[90] Zhu F, et al. Biomechanical responses of a pig head under blast loading: a computational simulation. Int J Numer Methods Biomed Eng 2013;29(3):392–407.

[91] Yarnell AM, et al. Blast traumatic brain injury in the rat using a blast overpressure model. Curr Protoc Neurosci 2013. Chapter 9: p. Unit 9.41.

[92] Risling M, et al. Mechanisms of blast induced brain injuries, experimental studies in rats. Neuroimage 2011;54(Suppl 1):S89–97.

[93] Reneer DV, et al. A multi-mode shock tube for investigation of blast-induced traumatic brain injury. J Neurotrauma 2011;28(1):95–104.

[94] Cernak I, et al. The pathobiology of blast injuries and blast-induced neurotrauma as identified using a new experimental model of injury in mice. Neurobiol Dis 2011;41(2):538–51.

[95] Chavko M, et al. Relationship between orientation to a blast and pressure wave propagation inside the rat brain. J Neurosci Methods 2011;195(1):61–6.

[96] Sundaramurthy A, et al. Blast-induced biomechanical loading of the rat: an experimental and anatomically accurate computational blast injury model. J Neurotrauma 2012;29(13):2352–64.

[97] Logsdon AF, et al. Low-intensity blast wave model for preclinical assessment of closed-head mild traumatic brain injury in rodents. J Vis Exp 2020;165.

[98] Unnikrishnan G, et al. Animal orientation affects brain biomechanical responses to blast-wave exposure. J Biomech Eng 2021;143(5).

[99] Sharpless SK, Halpern LM. The electrical excitability of chronically isolated cortex studied by means of permanently implanted electrodes. Electroencephalogr Clin Neurophysiol 1962;14:244–55.

[100] Timofeev I, et al. Origin of slow cortical oscillations in deafferented cortical slabs. Cereb Cortex 2000;10(12):1185–99.

[101] Topolnik L, Steriade M, Timofeev I. Partial cortical deafferentation promotes development of paroxysmal activity. Cereb Cortex 2003;13(8):883–93.

[102] Nita DA, et al. Increased propensity to seizures after chronic cortical deafferentation in vivo. J Neurophysiol 2006;95(2):902–13.

[103] Avramescu S, Timofeev I. Synaptic strength modulation after cortical trauma: a role in epileptogenesis. J Neurosci 2008;28(27):6760–72.

[104] Hoffman SN, Salin PA, Prince DA. Chronic neocortical epileptogenesis in vitro. J Neurophysiol 1994;71(5):1762–73.

[105] Salin P, et al. Axonal sprouting in layer V pyramidal neurons of chronically injured cerebral cortex. J Neurosci 1995;15(12):8234–45.

[106] Graber KD, Prince DA. Tetrodotoxin prevents posttraumatic epileptogenesis in rats. Ann Neurol 1999;46(2):234–42.

[107] Li H, Prince DA. Synaptic activity in chronically injured, epileptogenic sensory-motor neocortex. J Neurophysiol 2002;88(1):2–12.

[108] Li H, Bandrowski AE, Prince DA. Cortical injury affects short-term plasticity of evoked excitatory synaptic currents. J Neurophysiol 2005;93(1):146–56.

[109] Jin X, Huguenard JR, Prince DA. Impaired Cl- extrusion in layer V pyramidal neurons of chronically injured epileptogenic neocortex. J Neurophysiol 2005;93(4):2117–26.

[110] Jin X, Prince DA, Huguenard JR. Enhanced excitatory synaptic connectivity in layer v pyramidal neurons of chronically injured epileptogenic neocortex in rats. J Neurosci 2006;26(18):4891–900.

[111] Ping X, Jin X. Chronic posttraumatic epilepsy following neocortical undercut lesion in mice. PLoS One 2016;11(6), e0158231.

[112] Ping X, et al. Blocking receptor for advanced glycation end products (RAGE) or toll-like receptor 4 (TLR4) prevents posttraumatic epileptogenesis in mice. Epilepsia 2021;62(12):3105–16.

[113] Xiong W, et al. Preparing undercut model of posttraumatic epileptogenesis in rodents. J Vis Exp 2011;55.

[114] Ma X, et al. Animal models of traumatic brain injury and assessment of injury severity. Mol Neurobiol 2019;56(8):5332–45.

[115] Johnson VE, et al. Animal models of traumatic brain injury. Handb Clin Neurol 2015;127:115–28.

[116] Cernak I. Animal models of head trauma. NeuroRx 2005;2(3):410–22.

[117] McCutcheon V, et al. A novel model of traumatic brain injury in adult zebrafish demonstrates response to injury and treatment comparable with mammalian models. J Neurotrauma 2017;34(7):1382–93.

[118] Cho SJ, et al. Zebrafish model of posttraumatic epilepsy. Epilepsia 2020;61(8):1774–85.

[119] Saikumar J, et al. Inducing different severities of traumatic brain injury in Drosophila using a piezoelectric actuator. Nat Protoc 2021;16(1):263–82.

Chapter 7

Incidence of posttraumatic epilepsy in animal models of traumatic brain injury

Overview

Posttraumatic epilepsy (PTE) is a neurological consequence that develops over an unspecified latent period following traumatic brain injury (TBI). Posttraumatic seizures can be categorized by their occurrence after the initial injury into immediate (within 24 h), early (≤7 days), or late (>7 days) seizures, whereas late unprovoked spontaneous seizures are the hallmark of clinical PTE. In Chapter 6, we reviewed the six most widely used mechanical TBI animal models: fluid percussion injury, controlled cortical impact injury, weight drop injury, penetrating ballistic-like brain injury, blast-induced traumatic brain injury, and undercut injury. In this chapter, we will discuss which of these injuries lead to the development of PTE.

Fluid percussion injury

Fluid percussion injury (FPI) is one of the most used TBI animal models (Chapter 6). This model has been widely used in rats to investigate epilepsy. Inhibition [1], hyperexcitability [2–5], seizure susceptibility [6–9], and posttraumatic seizures in the early [10] and late phases are frequently studied.

In the FPI model, unprovoked spontaneous seizures generally occur several weeks following injury (Table 7.1). Several studies have reported low incidence from 0% to 3% [11–13], while others have documented a relatively high incidence of PTE. Three studies reported incidence of 27%–30% in rats 6–7 months postinjury [14–16]. Smith *et al.* demonstrated that 38% of rats developed PTE within 5 weeks. This is one of the shortest latencies observed in the FPI model; however, the mortality rate was exceptionally high (45%) [20]. PTE incidence of 43%–55% has been documented in three separate studies up to 12 months postinjury with a mortality rate up to 33% [17–19]. Kharatishvili *et al.* published a typical example of electrographic seizure that spread from the hippocampus to the cortex [17] (Fig. 7.1).

Posttraumatic Epilepsy. https://doi.org/10.1016/B978-0-323-90099-7.00003-4

TABLE 7.1 Summary of *in vivo* studies that have investigated posttraumatic epilepsy after traumatic brain injury.

TBI model	Species	Postinjury assessment (EEG)	Animals with epilepsy (%)	References
FPI	Rat	9 months	0%	[11]
FPI	Rat	11 months	0%	[12]
FPI	Mouse	6 months	3% (1/31)	[13]
FPI	Rat	6 months	27% (3/115)	[14]
FPI	Rat	Up to 6 months	30% (7/23)	[15]
FPI	Rat	Up to 189 days	30%	[16]
FPI	Rat	Up to 11 months Up to 12 months	50% (9/18) 43% (13/20)	[17]
FPI	Rat	Up to 52 weeks	50% (14/28)	[18]
FPI	Rat	8–21 weeks	55% (22/40)	[19]
FPI	Rat	2–5 weeks	37.5% (3/8)	[20]
CCI	Rat	4–11 months	13% (1/8)	[21]
CCI	Rat	Up to 619 days	20.3% (26/128)	[22]
CCI	Rat	Up to 14 days	43.7% (7/16)	[23]
CCI	Mouse	6 months	9% (4/45)	[13]
CCI	Mouse	Up to 16 weeks	50% (8/16)	[24]
CCI	Mouse	3.5 months 5 months	45% (8/18) 58% (11/18)	[25]
CCI	Mouse	42–71 days	20% (2/10) mild 36% (4/11) severe	[26]
CCI	Mouse	Up to 10 weeks	40% (12/30)	[27]
CCI	Mouse	Up to 90 days	28% (10/36)	[28]
CCI	Mouse	Up to 14 days Up to 30 days Up to 60 days Up to 90 days	13% (1/8) 20% (2/10) 27% (3/11) 14% (1/7)	[29]
WDI	Mouse	Up to 110 days	44% (4/9)	[30]
PBBI	Rat	1–6 months	7.5% (6/80)	[31]
PBBI	Rat	6 months	20% (4/20)	[31]
PBBI	Rat	6–11 months	Lesion only: 23% Lesion and copper: 96% Lesion and steel: 0%	[32]

TABLE 7.1 Summary of *in vivo* studies that have investigated posttraumatic epilepsy after traumatic brain injury—cont'd

TBI model	Species	Postinjury assessment (EEG)	Animals with epilepsy (%)	References
bTBI	Mouse	Up to 10 months	46% (6/13)	[33]
Undercut	Mouse	Up to 50 days Up to 90 days	33.3% (2/6) 62.5% (5/8)	[34]

bTBI, blast-induced traumatic brain injury; CCI, controlled cortical impact; EEG, electroencephalography; FPI, fluid percussion injury, PBBI: penetrating ballistic-like brain injury; WDI, weight drop injury.

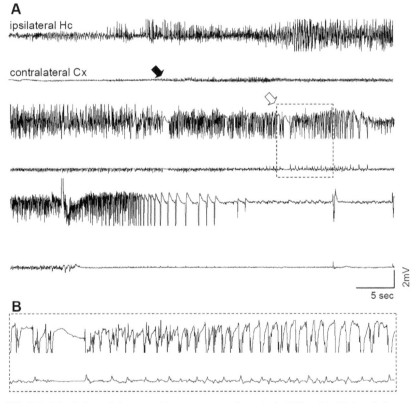

FIG. 7.1 Morphology of electrographic spontaneous seizures in the FPI model. (A) A typical example of a secondarily generalized tonic-clonic seizure that was recorded at 11 weeks postinjury. Seizure was first detected in the ipsilateral ventral hippocampus (Hc); from there, it spread after a short delay *(filled arrow)* to the contralateral parietal cortex (Cx). The duration of the seizure was 2 min 45 s. Electroencephalography (EEG) calibration bar is in the right lower corner of the panel. (B) EEG during a seizure at a higher temporal resolution (corresponds to dotted box in panel A). Note the typical spike-wave pattern. *(Reproduced with permission from Kharatishvili I, et al. A model of posttraumatic epilepsy induced by lateral fluid-percussion brain injury in rats. Neuroscience 2006;140(2):685–97.)*

Controlled cortical impact injury

The controlled cortical impact (CCI) injury model is widely used in epilepsy studies.

This model is frequently used due to its high reproducibility, high survivability after injury induction, and relative ease of use (Chapter 6). In addition to late posttraumatic seizures, the CCI model has also been used to determine abnormalities in evoked responses, sleep-wake states, excitability, and seizure susceptibility after injury [35–39].

The CCI model has successfully demonstrated unprovoked spontaneous seizures several weeks following induction of injury (Table 7.1). Studies involving rats reported 13%–44% incidence up to 619 days postinjury [21–23]. Mice are more frequently used to investigate PTE; however, posttraumatic seizures and incidence may be dependent on genetic background [40,41]. In particular, a study using C57/BL6 mice reported 9% incidence 6 months postinjury [13], while the incidence in CD1 mice was considerably higher, with 50%–58% incidence up to 5 months postinjury [24,25]. Hunt et al. documented incidence in varying injury severities. In mice with mild injury, the incidence was 20%; with severe injury, incidence was 36% 42–71 days postinjury [26]. The following year, the same group reported 40% incidence up to 10 weeks postinjury [27]. In 2020, Szu et al. published one study with 28% incidence up to 90 days postinjury [28] and another study characterizing incidence at 14, 30, 60, and 90 days postinjury with documented incidence of 13%, 20%, 27%, and 14%, respectively [29]. In this manuscript, representative examples of electrographic seizures were shown (Fig. 7.2). In 2021, Di Sapia et al. reported 45% incidence at 3.5 months and 58% incidence at 5 months postinjury [25]. Representative examples of electrographic seizures that occur bilaterally or unilaterally in the contralateral hemisphere were also shown (Fig. 7.3).

Weight drop injury

PTE studies involving the weight drop injury (WDI) model are nearly absent. The studies that utilized electroencephalography (EEG) investigated the immediate phase of TBI (within the first 2 h) [42], examined power spectral analysis [43], cortical spreading depolarization [44], and seizure susceptibility after injury [45–47]. Of the studies that used long-term EEG, vigilance states were analyzed rather than the occurrence of PTE [48,49]. To date, there is only one study with documented evidence of PTE. In 2019, Shandra et al. reported 44% incidence up to 110 days after triple impact using the Marmarou model [30].

Penetrating ballistic-like brain injury

The most commonly reported outcomes of penetrating ballistic-like brain injury (PBBI) are focused on the biological response to injury and neurological deficits. The studies that employed EEG targeted the early phase, within the first

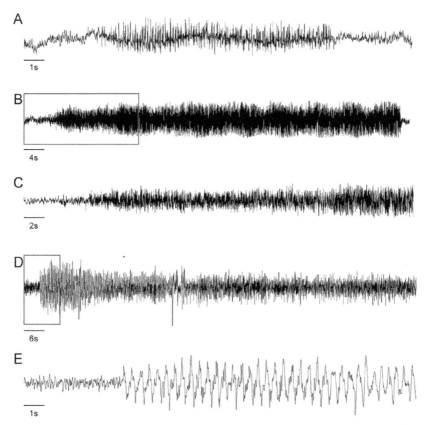

FIG. 7.2 Morphology of electrographic spontaneous seizures in the CCI model. (A) Typical spontaneous seizure with increased frequency and amplitude (fast polyspike) followed by return to baseline. (B) A seizure initiated from a ramp-up of baseline and developed into full seizure. (C) Expanded electroencephalography (EEG) from *red* boxed area in (B) demonstrating baseline gradually increasing in amplitude and progressing into a full seizure. (D) A seizure exhibiting 3 Hz spikes. (E) Expanded EEG from *red* boxed area in (D). *(Reproduced with permission from Szu JI, et al. Aquaporin-4 dysregulation in a controlled cortical impact injury model of posttraumatic epilepsy. Neuroscience 2020;428:140–53.)*

72 h after injury [50–52], while the use of long-term EEG to determine PTE incidence is sparse. Lu *et al.* reported 7.5% incidence in a ballistic-like injury in rats 1–6 months postinjury [31]. This same group also used a stainless steel ball projectile to induce injury in rats. PTE incidence of 20% was reported 6 months postinjury [31] (Table 7.1). Kendirli *et al.* documented posttraumatic seizures after penetrating stab wounds to the brain. In this study, PTE was reported in 23% with lesion only, 96% with lesion and copper, and 0% with lesion and stainless steel 6 and 7 months postinjury [32] (Table 7.1). To date, these are the only studies that have investigated PTE in this model.

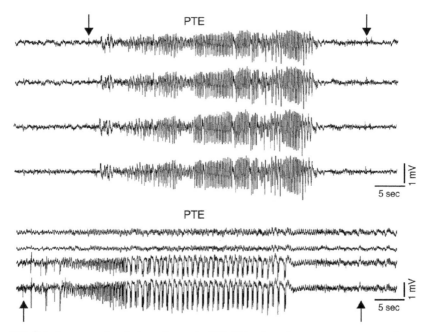

FIG. 7.3 Representative electrocorticography (ECoG) tracings of spontaneous recurrent seizures recorded in the CCI model. (A) ECoG seizures may occur bilaterally. (B) ECoG seizures may occur unilaterally in the contralateral hemisphere. *Black arrows* indicate the beginning and end of the seizure events. *(Reproduced with permission from Di Sapia R, et al. In-depth characterization of a mouse model of post-traumatic epilepsy for biomarker and drug discovery. Acta Neuropathol Commun 2021;9(1):76.)*

Blast-induced traumatic brain injury

Blast-induced traumatic brain injury (bTBI) has been studied for many years now; however, the occurrence of posttraumatic seizures is not generally assessed. The most commonly reported outcomes of bTBI are neuropathological and behavioral assessments, and the majority of studies do not involve EEG. In the studies that employed EEG, some used it as method to determine cerebral function after injury, such as depression of cortical activity [53–55], while other studies used EEG to examine changes in neural oscillation activity, frequency, amplitude, power spectral density, and evoked potentials after injury [56–59]. To date, the only documented PTE incidence was from a study involving a repetitive mild TBI in which incidence of 46% was reported after triple blast [33] (Table 7.1).

Undercut traumatic brain injury

This model has been frequently used in rodents to investigate neurophysiological mechanisms of posttraumatic epileptogenesis such as hyperexcitability

[60–62], field potentials [63–65], evoked responses [66,67], and seizure susceptibility [68]. Although this model has been used extensively, PTE studies are limited. Ping *et al.* reported 33% incidence of PTE at 50 days and 63% incidence 90 days postinjury. To date, this is the only study documenting PTE in this model [34] (Table 7.1).

In this chapter, we reviewed evidence for posttraumatic epilepsy in various TBI animal models. These studies have demonstrated the significance of EEG as a diagnostic tool to investigate epileptogenesis. Overall, considerable progress has been made in modeling epilepsy in rodents after mechanical TBI and most information about the neuropathological mechanisms of epileptogenesis has been derived from animal models; however, there is still a need for standardization. Standardization of species and genetic background, injury severity, video-EEG parameters, and spontaneous seizure criteria is urgently needed to identify relevant EEG characteristics that *consistently* indicate an injured and epileptic brain. Detailed evaluation of electrophysiological and histological abnormalities is crucial not only to determine the cellular and molecular changes underlying PTE, but also to define biomarkers for new therapeutic treatment development (Chapters 11 and 12).

References

[1] Reeves TM, et al. The effects of traumatic brain injury on inhibition in the hippocampus and dentate gyrus. Brain Res 1997;757(1):119–32.

[2] Lowenstein DH, et al. Selective vulnerability of dentate hilar neurons following traumatic brain injury: a potential mechanistic link between head trauma and disorders of the hippocampus. J Neurosci 1992;12(12):4846–53.

[3] Santhakumar V, et al. Granule cell hyperexcitability in the early post-traumatic rat dentate gyrus: the 'irritable mossy cell' hypothesis. J Physiol 2000;524(Pt 1):117–34.

[4] Santhakumar V, et al. Long-term hyperexcitability in the hippocampus after experimental head trauma. Ann Neurol 2001;50(6):708–17.

[5] Echegoyen J, et al. Single application of a CB1 receptor antagonist rapidly following head injury prevents long-term hyperexcitability in a rat model. Epilepsy Res 2009;85(1):123–7.

[6] Hamm RJ, et al. The effect of postinjury kindled seizures on cognitive performance of traumatically brain-injured rats. Exp Neurol 1995;136(2):143–8.

[7] Atkins CM, et al. Post-traumatic seizure susceptibility is attenuated by hypothermia therapy. Eur J Neurosci 2010;32(11):1912–20.

[8] Bao YH, et al. Post-traumatic seizures exacerbate histopathological damage after fluid-percussion brain injury. J Neurotrauma 2011;28(1):35–42.

[9] Mukherjee S, et al. Increased seizure susceptibility in mice 30 days after fluid percussion injury. Front Neurol 2013;4:28.

[10] Andrade P, et al. Acute non-convulsive status epilepticus after experimental traumatic brain injury in rats. J Neurotrauma 2019;36(11):1890–907.

[11] Hayward NM, et al. Association of chronic vascular changes with functional outcome after traumatic brain injury in rats. J Neurotrauma 2010;27(12):2203–19.

[12] Kharatishvili I, et al. Quantitative diffusion MRI of hippocampus as a surrogate marker for post-traumatic epileptogenesis. Brain 2007;130(Pt 12):3155–68.

[13] Bolkvadze T, Pitkanen A. Development of post-traumatic epilepsy after controlled cortical impact and lateral fluid-percussion-induced brain injury in the mouse. J Neurotrauma 2012;29(5):789–812.

[14] Lapinlampi N, et al. Postinjury weight rather than cognitive or behavioral impairment predicts development of posttraumatic epilepsy after lateral fluid-percussion injury in rats. Epilepsia 2020;61(9):2035–52.

[15] Shultz SR, et al. Can structural or functional changes following traumatic brain injury in the rat predict epileptic outcome? Epilepsia 2013;54(7):1240–50.

[16] Bragin A, et al. Pathologic electrographic changes after experimental traumatic brain injury. Epilepsia 2016;57(5):735–45.

[17] Kharatishvili I, et al. A model of posttraumatic epilepsy induced by lateral fluid-percussion brain injury in rats. Neuroscience 2006;140(2):685–97.

[18] Reid AY, et al. The progression of electrophysiologic abnormalities during epileptogenesis after experimental traumatic brain injury. Epilepsia 2016;57(10):1558–67.

[19] Li L, et al. Spatial and temporal profile of high-frequency oscillations in posttraumatic epileptogenesis. Neurobiol Dis 2021;161, 105544.

[20] Smith D, et al. Convulsive seizures and EEG spikes after lateral fluid-percussion injury in the rat. Epilepsy Res 2018;147:87–94.

[21] Statler KD, et al. A potential model of pediatric posttraumatic epilepsy. Epilepsy Res 2009;86(2–3):221–3.

[22] Kelly KM, et al. Posttraumatic seizures and epilepsy in adult rats after controlled cortical impact. Epilepsy Res 2015;117:104–16.

[23] Nichols J, et al. Traumatic brain injury induces rapid enhancement of cortical excitability in juvenile rats. CNS Neurosci Ther 2015;21(2):193–203.

[24] Guo D, et al. Rapamycin attenuates the development of posttraumatic epilepsy in a mouse model of traumatic brain injury. PLoS One 2013;8(5), e64078.

[25] Di Sapia R, et al. In-depth characterization of a mouse model of post-traumatic epilepsy for biomarker and drug discovery. Acta Neuropathol Commun 2021;9(1):76.

[26] Hunt RF, Scheff SW, Smith BN. Posttraumatic epilepsy after controlled cortical impact injury in mice. Exp Neurol 2009;215(2):243–52.

[27] Hunt RF, Scheff SW, Smith BN. Regionally localized recurrent excitation in the dentate gyrus of a cortical contusion model of posttraumatic epilepsy. J Neurophysiol 2010;103(3):1490–500.

[28] Szu JI, et al. Modulation of posttraumatic epileptogenesis in aquaporin-4 knockout mice. Epilepsia 2020;61(7):1503–14.

[29] Szu JI, et al. Aquaporin-4 dysregulation in a controlled cortical impact injury model of posttraumatic epilepsy. Neuroscience 2020;428:140–53.

[30] Shandra O, et al. Repetitive diffuse mild traumatic brain injury causes an atypical astrocyte response and spontaneous recurrent seizures. J Neurosci 2019;39(10):1944–63.

[31] Lu XM, et al. Post-traumatic epilepsy and seizure susceptibility in rat models of penetrating and closed-head brain injury. J Neurotrauma 2020;37(2):236–47.

[32] Kendirli MT, Rose DT, Bertram EH. A model of posttraumatic epilepsy after penetrating brain injuries: effect of lesion size and metal fragments. Epilepsia 2014;55(12):1969–77.

[33] Bugay V, et al. A mouse model of repetitive blast traumatic brain injury reveals post-trauma seizures and increased neuronal excitability. J Neurotrauma 2020;37(2):248–61.

[34] Ping X, Jin X. Chronic posttraumatic epilepsy following neocortical undercut lesion in mice. PLoS One 2016;11(6), e0158231.

[35] Yang L, et al. Spontaneous epileptiform activity in rat neocortex after controlled cortical impact injury. J Neurotrauma 2010;27(8):1541–8.

[36] Konduru SS, et al. Sleep-wake characteristics in a mouse model of severe traumatic brain injury: relation to posttraumatic epilepsy. Epilepsia Open 2021;6(1):181–94.

[37] Koenig JB, et al. Glycolytic inhibitor 2-deoxyglucose prevents cortical hyperexcitability after traumatic brain injury. JCI Insight 2019;5.

[38] Cantu D, et al. In vivo KPT-350 treatment decreases cortical hyperexcitability following traumatic brain injury. Brain Inj 2020;34(11):1489–96.

[39] Carver CM, et al. Blockade of TRPC channels limits cholinergic-driven hyperexcitability and seizure susceptibility after traumatic brain injury. Front Neurosci 2021;15, 681144.

[40] Ferraro TN, et al. Mapping loci for pentylenetetrazol-induced seizure susceptibility in mice. J Neurosci 1999;19(16):6733–9.

[41] McKhann II GM, et al. Mouse strain differences in kainic acid sensitivity, seizure behavior, mortality, and hippocampal pathology. Neuroscience 2003;122(2):551–61.

[42] Nilsson P, et al. Epileptic seizure activity in the acute phase following cortical impact trauma in rat. Brain Res 1994;637(1–2):227–32.

[43] Ucar T, et al. Modified experimental mild traumatic brain injury model. J Trauma 2006;60(3):558–65.

[44] Aboghazleh R, et al. Brainstem and cortical spreading depolarization in a closed head injury rat model. Int J Mol Sci 2021;22(21).

[45] Golarai G, et al. Physiological and structural evidence for hippocampal involvement in persistent seizure susceptibility after traumatic brain injury. J Neurosci 2001;21(21):8523–37.

[46] Efendioglu M, et al. Combination therapy of gabapentin and N-acetylcysteine against posttraumatic epilepsy in rats. Neurochem Res 2020;45(8):1802–12.

[47] Ghadiri T, et al. Neuronal injury and death following focal mild brain injury: the role of network excitability and seizure. Iran J Basic Med Sci 2020;23(1):63–70.

[48] Buchele F, et al. Novel rat model of weight drop-induced closed diffuse traumatic brain injury compatible with electrophysiological recordings of vigilance states. J Neurotrauma 2016;33(13):1171–80.

[49] Sabir M, et al. Impact of traumatic brain injury on sleep structure, electrocorticographic activity and transcriptome in mice. Brain Behav Immun 2015;47:118–30.

[50] Williams AJ, et al. Characterization of a new rat model of penetrating ballistic brain injury. J Neurotrauma 2005;22(2):313–31.

[51] Lu XC, et al. Electrocortical pathology in a rat model of penetrating ballistic-like brain injury. J Neurotrauma 2011;28(1):71–83.

[52] Lu XC, et al. Similarities and differences of acute nonconvulsive seizures and other epileptic activities following penetrating and ischemic brain injuries in rats. J Neurotrauma 2013;30(7):580–90.

[53] Axelsson H, et al. Physiological changes in pigs exposed to a blast wave from a detonating high-explosive charge. Mil Med 2000;165(2):119–26.

[54] Chen HJ, et al. An open air research study of blast-induced traumatic brain injury to goats. Chin J Traumatol 2015;18(5):267–74.

[55] Li BC, et al. Blast-induced traumatic brain injury of goats in confined space. Neurol Res 2014;36(11):974–82.

[56] Liu Y, et al. Abnormalities in dynamic brain activity caused by mild traumatic brain injury are partially rescued by the cannabinoid type-2 receptor inverse agonist SMM-189. eNeuro 2017;4(4).

[57] Cernak I. The importance of systemic response in the pathobiology of blast-induced neurotrauma. Front Neurol 2010;1:151.

[58] Chen C, et al. Quantitative electroencephalography in a swine model of blast-induced brain injury. Brain Inj 2017;31(1):120–6.

[59] Ordek G, et al. Electrophysiological correlates of blast-wave induced cerebellar injury. Sci Rep 2018;8(1):13633.

[60] Prince DA, Tseng GF. Epileptogenesis in chronically injured cortex: in vitro studies. J Neurophysiol 1993;69(4):1276–91.

[61] Hoffman SN, Salin PA, Prince DA. Chronic neocortical epileptogenesis in vitro. J Neurophysiol 1994;71(5):1762–73.

[62] Li H, Prince DA. Synaptic activity in chronically injured, epileptogenic sensory-motor neocortex. J Neurophysiol 2002;88(1):2–12.

[63] Topolnik L, Steriade M, Timofeev I. Partial cortical deafferentation promotes development of paroxysmal activity. Cereb Cortex 2003;13(8):883–93.

[64] Nita DA, et al. Increased propensity to seizures after chronic cortical deafferentation in vivo. J Neurophysiol 2006;95(2):902–13.

[65] Avramescu S, Timofeev I. Synaptic strength modulation after cortical trauma: a role in epileptogenesis. J Neurosci 2008;28(27):6760–72.

[66] Li H, Bandrowski AE, Prince DA. Cortical injury affects short-term plasticity of evoked excitatory synaptic currents. J Neurophysiol 2005;93(1):146–56.

[67] Jin X, Prince DA, Huguenard JR. Enhanced excitatory synaptic connectivity in layer v pyramidal neurons of chronically injured epileptogenic neocortex in rats. J Neurosci 2006;26(18):4891–900.

[68] Ping X, et al. Blocking receptor for advanced glycation end products (RAGE) or toll-like receptor 4 (TLR4) prevents posttraumatic epileptogenesis in mice. Epilepsia 2021;62(12):3105–16.

Chapter 8

Cellular and molecular changes in animal models of posttraumatic epilepsy

Overview

Posttraumatic epilepsy (PTE) is acquired after initial traumatic brain injury (TBI) leading to unprovoked spontaneous recurrent seizures. In Chapter 7, we reviewed PTE incidence in six mechanical TBI animal models most widely used in preclinical research. Each animal model has demonstrated evidence of PTE, whether from a single injury (fluid percussion injury, controlled cortical impact injury, penetrating ballistic-like injury, and undercut injury) or multiple injuries (repeated weight drop injury and repeated blast-induced injury). In this chapter, we examine the cellular and molecular changes observed in animals that develop PTE *vs*. animals that do not develop PTE after TBI.

Mossy fiber sprouting

Mossy fiber sprouting (sprouting of the "mossy fiber" axons of the dentate granule cells in the hippocampus) is an example of a permanent change in anatomy and connectivity that can result from TBI. The degree of sprouting is usually indicative of injury severity and can be observed in humans with TBI [1,2]. This phenomenon has been documented in animal models of epilepsy [3] as well as TBI studies such as lateral fluid percussion injury (LFPI) and controlled cortical impact (CCI) injury [4,5]. Kharatishvili *et al.* reported significantly denser mossy fiber sprouting in rats that developed PTE by 12 months post-LFPI than in rats that did not develop epilepsy. Sprouting was also denser ipsilateral to the injury than contralateral [6] (Fig. 8.1). This report suggests that the degree of mossy fiber sprouting after injury may be predictive of the development of PTE.

Reactive astrocytes

Not surprisingly, reactive astrocytosis has been reported in both animal and human studies of posttraumatic epilepsy (PTE). Gliosis was observed in neocortical tissue specimens collected from patients with head trauma and is considered

Posttraumatic Epilepsy. https://doi.org/10.1016/B978-0-323-90099-7.00005-8

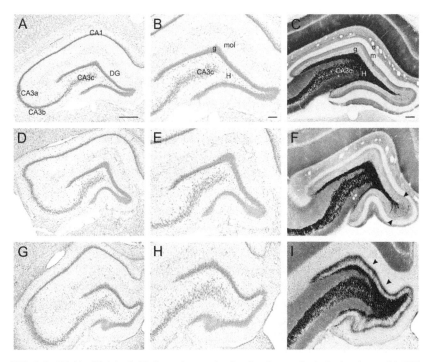

FIG. 8.1 Digitized bright-field photomicrographs showing damage in the brain of rats with PTE as a consequence of lateral fluid percussion injury (LFPI). (A) A Thionin-stained section from the septal end of the hippocampus in a control rat. (B) Same section, the dentate gyrus at higher magnification. (C) An adjacent Timm-stained section from a control rat showing the normal distribution of mossy fibers. (D) A Thionin-stained section from the septal end of the hippocampus in a rat with LFPI 10 months after the injury. (E) Same section, the dentate gyrus at higher magnification. Note the loss of hilar cells compared with the control animal in panel A. (F) An adjacent Timm-stained section from a rat with FPI. Note the sparse labeling of mossy fibers in the inner molecular layer of the dentate gyrus *(black arrows)*. (G) A Thionin-stained section from the septal end of the hippocampus in a rat with LFPI that developed epilepsy 12 months after the injury. (H) Same section, the dentate gyrus at higher magnification. Note the loss of hilar neurons compared with the LFPI animal in panel E. (I) An adjacent Timm-stained section from an animal with LFPI that developed epilepsy. Note dense mossy fiber sprouting *(black arrows)*. Abbreviations: DG, dentate gyrus; g, granule cell layer; h, hilus; i, inner molecular layer; mol, molecular layer; m, midmolecular layer; o, outer molecular layer. Scale bar = 100 μm in panels B, C, E, F, H, I. Scale bar = 1 mm in panels A, D, G. *(Reproduced with permission from Kharatishvili I, et al. A model of posttraumatic epilepsy induced by lateral fluid-percussion brain injury in rats. Neuroscience 2006;140(2):685–97.)*

a risk factor for epilepsy [1]. Shandra *et al.* correlated glutamate transporter-1 (GLT-1) expression loss with atypical astrocytes in a repeated weight drop injury model [7]. Mice that developed PTE had significant increases in GLT-1 expression and greater GLT-1 area loss fractions compared with mice that did not develop PTE 110 days postinjury [7]. This study suggests that a specific phenotype of reactive astrocytes appears to be associated with the development of PTE.

Aquaporin-4 dysregulation and mislocalization

Astrocyte molecules play critical roles in the development of epilepsy [8]. Specifically, alterations in the astrocytic water channel aquaporin-4 (AQP4) have been shown in preclinical models of epilepsy and traumatic brain injury (TBI) [9,10]. Szu *et al.* detected significant AQP4 upregulation in the ipsilateral frontal cortex and hippocampus in mice that developed PTE compared with nonepileptic mice [11]. Mislocalization of AQP4 was detected in the frontal cortex of PTE mice at 14 days postinjury (Fig. 8.2). In PTE mice, hippocampal AQP4 dysregulation was also observed primarily at 14 days postinjury at which time AQP4 immunoreactivity was largely expressed in the soma and major processes of astrocytes, while blood vessels lacked perivascular AQP4 expression [11]. These findings suggest that AQP4 dysregulation may contribute to the pathogenesis of PTE (Chapter 12).

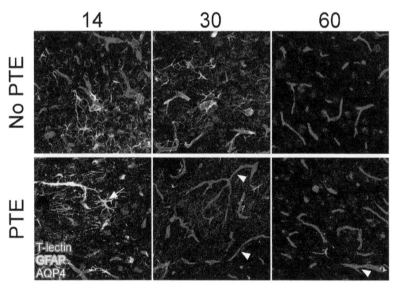

FIG. 8.2 Mislocalization of AQP4 in the frontal cortex of mice with PTE in a CCI animal model. In mice without PTE (top), AQP4 is partially redistributed. Specifically, loss of perivascular AQP4 is detected in the frontal cortex of mice without PTE at 14 days postinjury (*red*-colored blood vessels showing lack of AQP4 colocalization); however, a partial recovery of perivascular AQP4 is observed at 30 and 60 days postinjury (*magenta*-colored blood vessels indicating colocalization with perivascular AQP4). In mice with PTE (bottom), mislocalization of AQP4 is observed at 14 days postinjury (*white arrow*, cyan color showing colocalization of AQP4 *(blue)* with astrocyte (GFAP, *green*)), while AQP4 mislocalization is less prominent at 30 and 60 days postinjury with some vessels devoid of AQP4 (*white arrowhead* on blood vessels (T-lectin)). AQP4: aquaporin-4, GFAP: glial fibrillary acidic protein, T-lectin: tomato lectin, CCI: controlled cortical impact. *(Reproduced with permission from Szu JI, et al. Aquaporin-4 dysregulation in a controlled cortical impact injury model of posttraumatic epilepsy. Neuroscience 2020;428:140–53.)*

Despite the fact that the development of PTE after TBI is clinically accepted, the pathophysiology by which trauma leads to spontaneous seizures is still unknown. Clinically relevant models of PTE are key to understanding the molecular and cellular mechanisms underlying the development of PTE. In this chapter, we reviewed the cellular and molecular changes observed in animals that developed PTE compared to animals that did not develop PTE after TBI. What is quite remarkable upon review of this field is that most animal TBI studies with evidence of PTE characterized seizure occurrence (Chapter 7) but did not conduct detailed cellular and molecular analysis comparing PTE *vs.* non-PTE animals. While it is important to study changes between injured and uninjured animals (thereby elucidating cellular and molecular cascades after TBI), it is even more critical to investigate cellular and molecular differences between PTE animals and non-PTE animals *controlling for TBI*. Only this comparison will further our understanding of the *unique* cellular and molecular mechanisms underlying PTE.

References

[1] Swartz BE, et al. Hippocampal cell loss in posttraumatic human epilepsy. Epilepsia 2006;47(8):1373–82.

[2] Mathern GW, et al. The pathogenic and progressive features of chronic human hippocampal epilepsy. Epilepsy Res 1996;26(1):151–61.

[3] Cavarsan CF, et al. Is mossy fiber sprouting a potential therapeutic target for epilepsy? Front Neurol 2018;9:1023.

[4] Santhakumar V, et al. Long-term hyperexcitability in the hippocampus after experimental head trauma. Ann Neurol 2001;50(6):708–17.

[5] Hunt RF, Scheff SW, Smith BN. Posttraumatic epilepsy after controlled cortical impact injury in mice. Exp Neurol 2009;215(2):243–52.

[6] Kharatishvili I, et al. A model of posttraumatic epilepsy induced by lateral fluid-percussion brain injury in rats. Neuroscience 2006;140(2):685–97.

[7] Shandra O, et al. Repetitive diffuse mild traumatic brain injury causes an atypical astrocyte response and spontaneous recurrent seizures. J Neurosci 2019;39(10):1944–63.

[8] Hubbard JA, Binder DK. Astrocytes and epilepsy. Elsevier: Academic Press; 2016.

[9] Binder DK, Nagelhus EA, Ottersen OP. Aquaporin-4 and epilepsy. Glia 2012;60(8):1203–14.

[10] Binder DK. Astrocytes: stars of the sacred disease. Epilepsy Curr 2018;18(3):172–9.

[11] Szu JI, et al. Aquaporin-4 dysregulation in a controlled cortical impact injury model of posttraumatic epilepsy. Neuroscience 2020;428:140–53.

Chapter 9

Blood-brain barrier disruption and posttraumatic epilepsy

Overview

The blood-brain barrier (BBB) acts as both a physical and a physiological barrier between circulating blood and the central nervous system (CNS). The BBB is composed of specialized cell populations that tightly regulate both the influx and the efflux of ions, molecules, and peripheral cells to maintain CNS homeostasis. The endothelial cells of the BBB interact with mural cells, immune cells, and glial cells as a "neurovascular unit" to perform critical functions, and disturbances of these barrier functions are an important component in the manifestation of neurological disease [1]. BBB integrity can be compromised due to primary damage to the microvasculature, which can be a result of blunt (nonpenetrating), penetrating, and blast-induced traumatic brain injury (TBI) [2]. BBB breakdown can cause edema and an increase in intracranial pressure, resulting in secondary brain injury following TBI. Secondary brain injury can lead to the manifestation of seizures months to years following the initial trauma. Although epidemiological studies have demonstrated a clear relationship between injury severity and the likelihood of developing epilepsy following trauma, evidence also suggests an important role of BBB permeability in epileptogenesis. Preclinical models have demonstrated that prolonged opening of the BBB can lead to the development of epilepsy, and recurring seizures can lead to disturbances in BBB integrity; therefore, identifying markers of BBB disruption is crucial in the early identification and treatment of posttraumatic epilepsy (PTE). In this chapter, we will discuss the current understanding of BBB disruption in PTE, evaluate how BBB dysfunction following TBI may lead to the progression of epilepsy, and consider whether disturbances in the BBB can be used as a predictive factor for early identification of PTE.

Blood-brain barrier permeability in traumatic brain injury

The BBB was first described by Paul Ehrlich in the 1800s. Following intravenous injection of water-soluble aniline dyes into the systemic circulation, the dye could be observed throughout most tissues but not in the CNS [3]. A few years later, Goldmann concluded that dyes injected into the systemic circulation are observed

Posttraumatic Epilepsy. https://doi.org/10.1016/B978-0-323-90099-7.00015-0

in all tissues except the brain and spinal cord. Conversely, dye injected into the cerebrospinal fluid (CSF) stained the brain but was not found in peripheral tissues [4,5]. These studies paved the way for our current understanding of the tightly regulated restrictive nature of the BBB. In 1992, Povlishock demonstrated that moderate TBI in rats increased vascular permeability to serum albumin throughout the cortex and underlying hippocampi [6]. Subsequently, Halley showed that after mild TBI using a fluid percussion injury (FPI) device, the protein tracer horseradish peroxidase (HRP), injected intravenously, can be detected in multiple regions rostral and caudal of the injury site in cortical and subcortical regions [7]. BBB breakdown and increased "leakiness" of the BBB following TBI are recapitulated in multiple preclinical studies [8–11]. Following TBI, lasting BBB breakdown may contribute to the onset of epileptogenesis [12] (Fig. 9.1).

In preclinical models, long-term BBB disruption may contribute to the development of epileptiform activity. The contrast agent gadobutrol (Gd) can be used to quantify BBB permeability in rats following injury using magnetic resonance imaging (MRI) [13,14]. Following induction of lateral FPI in rats, Gd-contrast enhancement is most evident in the perilesional cortex 4 days postinjury and can be observed up to 10 months following brain injury [13]. The presence of serum albumin in the brain extracellular space due to BBB disruption has been suggested to lead to hyperexcitability and may contribute to the development of epilepsy following injury [15,16]. Exposing rat cortices to albumin leads to hypersynchronized epileptiform activity 1 week following exposure that is indistinguishable to that of rats treated with the BBB-disrupting agent deoxycholic acid sodium salt suggesting that the presence of serum albumin in the brain could lead to hyperexcitability [15]. Epileptiform activity is also induced in rats that are exposed to native serum and denatured serum suggesting that CNS exposure to serum proteins could lead to hyperexcitability following BBB disruption (Fig. 9.2). Friedman also reported that following BBB disruption serum albumin is taken up by astrocytes through transforming growth factor-beta (TGF-β), a pleiotropic cytokine, leading to impairment in K^+ buffering prior to the onset of epileptiform activity [17]. Albumin taken up by astrocytes binds and activates TGF-β signaling which can elicit multiple responses including impairment of K^+ buffering and degradation of perineuronal nets around inhibitory neurons [16,18].

One hypothesis suggests that elevated extracellular potassium could contribute to posttraumatic hyperexcitability and seizures [19]. Following FPI in rats, loss of inwardly-rectifying K^+ currents is observed in hippocampal glial cells 2 days postinjury which could contribute to early abnormal neuronal function [19]. Abnormal K^+ buffering could be due to a downregulation in Kir4.1, the major inwardly rectifying potassium channel expressed in astrocytes, which is observed 24 h following treatment with the BBB-disrupting agent deoxycholic acid sodium salt compared to control rat cortices [16] (Fig. 9.3). Ivens *et al.* suggested that abnormal K^+ buffering following exposure to deoxycholic acid sodium salt is due to a transcriptional downregulation of Kir4.1 channels, but further studies are needed to confirm that these two events share a causal rela-

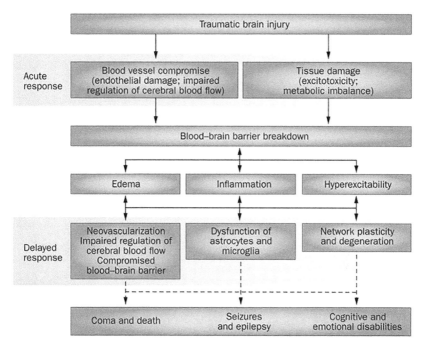

FIG. 9.1 Pathophysiological events in traumatic brain injury. Early symptoms of blood vessel and brain parenchyma compromise appear as blood flow irregularities and lead to metabolic imbalance, ischemia, hypoxia, and excitotoxicity. Such processes, which are associated with breakdown of the blood-brain barrier, might lead directly to the induction of signaling cascades and complex interactions between pathological processes within the neurovascular unit. The result of these interactions is the formation of brain edema, a local inflammatory response, and an increase in neuronal excitability. These early events might progress, interact, and initiate acute complications, such as increased intracranial pressure, ischemic cell damage, seizures, and death. In parallel, slower pathophysiological mechanisms, such as neovascularization, transformation and dysfunction of astrocytes, and changes in synaptic wiring, underlie the development of epilepsy, psychiatric, and cognitive disabilities, and neurodegenerative pathologies such as Alzheimer's disease. *(Reproduced with permission from Shlosberg D, et al. Blood-brain barrier breakdown as a therapeutic target in traumatic brain injury. Nat Rev Neurol 2010;6(7):393–403.)*

tionship with one another. Likewise, following FPI in rats, astrocyte potassium buffering impairment persists chronically in the neocortex but not hippocampus while mislocalization of Kir4.1 channels can also be observed at chronic time points in cortical but not hippocampal astrocytes [20] (Fig. 9.4). Conversely, animal studies have shown that the increase in extracellular K^+ that occurs following traumatic injury recovers within a few hours [21,22]. Following FPI in rats, resting K^+ and K^+ clearance is not impaired, but the larger K^+ increase observed was evoked as a consequence of neuronal activity suggesting regulation of K^+ is a consequence of injury rather than a mechanism responsible for posttraumatic excitability [23]. Following controlled cortical impact (CCI) injury, hippocampal and cortical protein levels of Kir4.1 are not significantly different in mice that develop PTE compared to mice that do not [24]. The inconsistencies between

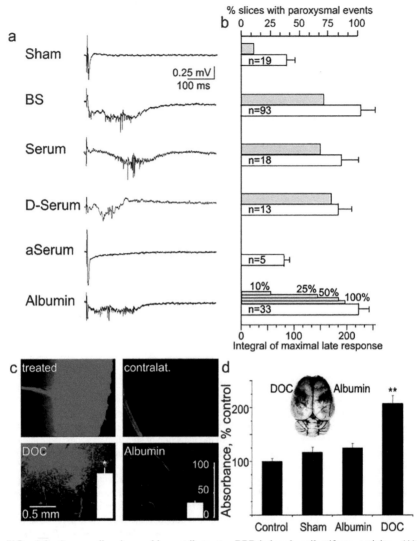

FIG. 9.2 Serum albumin could contribute to BBB-induced epileptiform activity. (A) Somatosensory cortex was perfused with artificial cerebrospinal fluid (sham), bile salts (BS), serum, denatured serum (D-Serum), electrolytic solution with serum concentrations (aSerum), and serum albumin in increasing concentrations (Albumin). Representative traces from extracellular recordings 7 day after treatment are displayed. (B) Quantification of the averaged integral of the late evoked responses in all slices *(white bars)* and percentage of slices in which paroxysmal activity was observed *(gray bars)*. Albumin concentrations (100% represents serum levels) are noted. *n* refers to the number of slices examined under each experimental condition. (C) Focal perfusion of albumin-Evans blue solution resulted in penetration of the albumin into the cortex of the ipsilateral (treated) hemisphere. In a different experiment, after intraperitoneal injection of Evans blue, extravasation of fluorescent albumin was more prominent in the deoxycholic acid (DOC)-treated compared with the albumin-treated hemisphere. The *white bars* represent averaged color intensity values (*n* = 20 sections in each experiment). (D) Photometric quantification of Evans blue-albumin brain concentrations in nontreated (control), sham-operated, albumin and DOC-treated brains. Note that only DOC treatment caused a significant increase in dye penetration. Inset, Brain after bilateral cranial window operation and intraperitoneal Evans blue injection. The right hemisphere was perfused with albumin and the left with DOC. *P < .05; **P < .01. *(Reproduced with permission from Seiffert E, et al. Lasting blood-brain barrier disruption induces epileptic focus in the rat somatosensory cortex. J Neurosci 2004;24(36):7829–836.)*

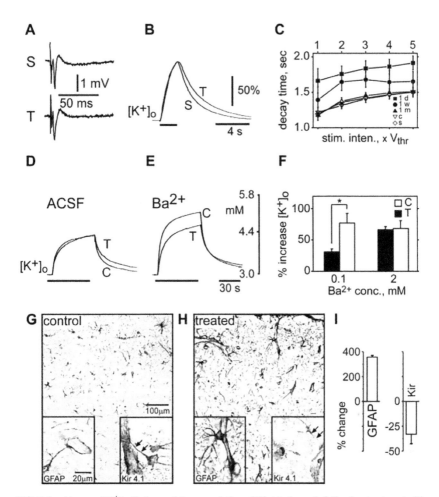

FIG. 9.3 Abnormal K^+ buffering and downregulation of Kir4.1 channels following treatment with the BBB-disrupting agent deoxycholic acid sodium salt. (A) Representative traces showing normal evoked field potentials recorded 24 h after treatment in sham-operated (S) and treated (T) cortices. (B) Two superimposed traces of the $[K^+]_o$ signals in response to a 2 s, 25 Hz stimulation (marked as underlying bar). $[K^+]_o$ signals were normalized to maximal increase (100%, 4.34 and 4.84 mM for control and treated, respectively). (C) $[K^+]_o$ decay time to 50% of its maximal value 1 day (1d), 1 week (1w), and 1 month (1 m) after treatment as well as 1 day after sham-operation (s) and in non-operated controls (c) ($n=11, 2, 4, 7$, and 15, respectively). (D) and (E) Representative traces showing the effect of Ba^{2+} on ionophoretically induced $[K^+]_o$ increase in treated and control slices before (D) and after (E) addition of 0.1 mM Ba^{2+}. (F) Summary of Ba^{2+} effect on $[K^+]_o$ increase. (G) and (H) Images of glial fibrillary acidic protein (GFAP) immunostaining in cortical sections 24 h after treatment compared with controls. Insets: higher magnifications of GFAP (left) and Kir4.1 (right) immunostaining in consecutive sections from the same brain. Note the enhanced GFAP and reduced Kir immunostaining in morphologically identified astrocytes. Black arrows point to astrocyte processes toward neighboring vessels. (I) % change in mRNA levels for GFAP and Kir4.1 in albumin or DOC-treated cortices compared with the contralateral, nontreated hemisphere ($n=5$ for each group). *(Reproduced with permission from Ivens S, et al. TGF-beta receptor-mediated albumin uptake into astrocytes is involved in neocortical epileptogenesis, Brain 2007;130(Pt 2):535–47.)*

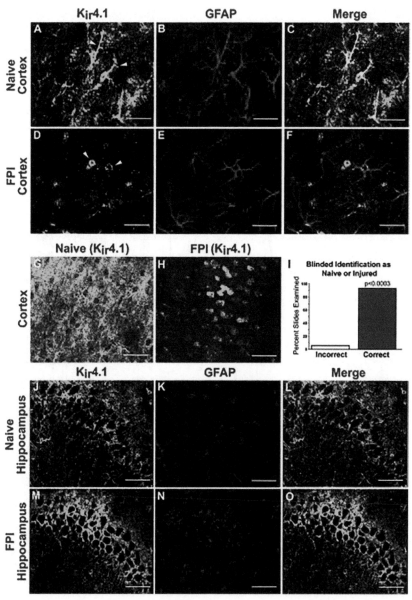

FIG. 9.4 FPI induces chronic Kir4.1 mislocalization in cortical but not hippocampal astrocytes. Confocal microscopic images of Kir4.1 *(green)* and GFAP *(red)* immunofluorescence were obtained from regions of neocortex (A–H) and CA3 hippocampus (J–O), corresponding to the regions from which astroglial patch-clamp recordings were obtained. Controls are shown in (A–C), (G), and (J–L). Sections obtained at 1 month after FPI are shown in (D–F), (H), and (M–O). (G, H), and all right-most images are merged images showing both Kir4.1 and GFAP immunoreactivity. (A–C) Naïve control cortex. Kir4.1 was expressed prominently in GFAP-positive astrocytic processes (arrowheads), as well as in astrocytic cell bodies. (D–F) Perilesional rostral parasagittal fluid percussion injury (rpFPI) cortex 1 month after injury. Compared with controls, Kir4.1 immunoreactivity in injured cortical

(Continued)

studies on whether Kir4.1 downregulation could contribute to the development of PTE following injury may be related to variability in models used, temporal differences, and spatial differences [16,20,24]. Taken together, these data suggest that K^+ homeostasis is altered in posttraumatic hyperexcitability, but further studies are needed to determine whether impaired K^+ buffering is a primary mechanism for seizure development following injury to the CNS.

Chronic BBB dysfunction can also be observed in patients with PTE. BBB function/dysfunction can be monitored in patients following TBI using the CSF/serum-albumin quotient (Q_A) by measuring albumin levels in the serum and CSF collected simultaneously. $Q_A \leq 0.007$ reflects normal BBB permeability in adults while a damaged or open BBB is defined as mild $(Q_A = 0.007–0.01)$ with further increases in Q_A correlated to TBI severity [25,26]. In patients, elevated Q_A can be observed up to 5 days post-TBI [27]. Following status epilepticus, patients also have elevated Q_A suggesting that BBB integrity is also compromised either preceding or following ictal events [28]. A less invasive approach to measure BBB integrity in patients following TBI is to use MRI. Images are collected before and after the peripheral administration of the contrast medium gadolinium-DTPA (Gd-DTPA) to evaluate BBB integrity. When using MRI to evaluate BBB disruption in 32 head trauma patients, increased BBB permeability was found in 77% of patients that developed PTE compared with 33% of patients without epilepsy suggesting that lasting BBB disruption may be causally related to the development of epilepsy following injury [29] (Fig. 9.5). In a subsequent study, approximately 80% of patients with PTE have BBB disruption compared to only 25% of nonepileptic patients [30]. Human autopsy of patients with a history of TBI reveals albumin and iron deposits in the perilesional cortex and thalamus which could be caused by BBB disruption [13]. Multiple studies have shown that BBB disruption can occur days before the onset of epileptiform activity, suggesting it could be used as a biomarker to predict seizure onset [15,31]. Following mild TBI, abnormal cortical activity is localized mainly to areas of BBB disruption in patients, suggesting a relationship between BBB leakage and epileptiform activity [29].

FIG. 9.4, CONT'D astrocytes (D–F) appears more prominent in swollen-appearing astrocytic cell bodies (arrowheads), whereas Kir4.1 immunoreactivity in GFAP-positive processes was markedly reduced. (G and H) Lower-magnification images of naïve (G) and injured cortex (H) similarly show that FPI was associated with an apparent loss of Kir4.1 immunoreactivity in finely ramifying processes. (I) Results of a histological analysis carried out under double-blind conditions that confirmed that the patterns of Kir4.1 expression in the somata and processes of astrocytes (D, F, and H) were distinct in naive and perilesional FPI neocortices. P=exact binomial probability. (J–O). in contrast to the injury-induced Kir4.1 mislocalization observed in neocortex, the expression pattern of Kir4.1 in the CA3 region of hippocampus of injured rats 30 days after injury (M–O) was comparable to controls (J–L). Scale bars: C, F, L, and O: 50 μm; G and H: 100 μm. *(Reproduced with permission from Stewart TH, et al. Chronic dysfunction of astrocytic inwardly rectifying K+ channels specific to the neocortical epileptic focus after fluid percussion injury in the rat. J Neurophysiol 2010;104(6):3345–360.)*

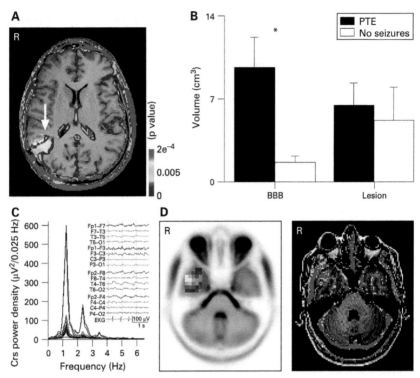

FIG. 9.5 Increased BBB disruption in patients with PTE. (A) Statistically significant enhancement of T1-weighted MRI scan in the region surrounding the cortical lesion in patient no 21, 10 days following the trauma. (B) Among patients with PTE, the volume of BBB disruption was significantly larger than that of nonepileptic patients. (C) A 34-year-old patient with PTE 1-month following mild TBI. Power spectrum showing a marked increase in power at 1.125 Hz, taken from an electroencephalography recording, demonstrating abnormal slowing maximal at right frontal and temporal electrodes (inset). (D) Standardized low-resolution brain electromagnetic tomography (sLORETA) localizing the pathological signal to the anterior parts of the right middle temporal gyrus (Brodmann area 21, left), and MRI signal enhancement indicating increased BBB permeability localized to the same region (right). $* = P < .05$. *(Reproduced with permission from Tomkins O, et al. Blood-brain barrier disruption in posttraumatic epilepsy. J Neurol Neurosurg Psychiatry 2008;79(7):774–77.)*

The BBB acts as the gatekeeper to the CNS and is important for brain homeostasis. Candidate mechanisms linking BBB disruption to abnormal neuronal firing include extravasation of K^+, albumin, or immune cells [15,32,33]. Cortical exposure to interferon-alpha (IFN-α), another cytokine with various functions, could also be a potential mechanism involved in hyperexcitability through disruption of the BBB. Exposing rat cortical slices to IFN-α leads to delayed epileptiform activity in $> 80\%$ of slices [34]. Generalized seizures have been reported in patients during IFN-α infusion, a therapy used for chronic viral hepatitis which may be due to BBB disruption [35,36]. These data suggest that leakage of the BBB and subsequent activation of neuroinflammatory processes could contribute to PTE which will be further discussed in Chapter 10.

Edema and posttraumatic epilepsy

Cerebral edema is a secondary injury that can result from TBI. Edema can occur by two basic mechanisms: vasogenic edema and cytotoxic edema [37–40]. Vasogenic edema is caused by a disruption in BBB integrity which leads to an uncontrolled influx of ions and proteins into the interstitial brain compartments, followed by fluid accumulation from the intravascular spaces, while cytotoxic edema occurs when cells swell as a result of a change in pH and ionic concentrations including potassium, sodium, and chloride [41]. Following TBI, cerebral edema occurs as a result of both vasogenic and cytotoxic mechanisms [37]. Cytotoxic edema following brain injury is associated with an increase in neuronal and glial volume. Cell volume increases from the influx of ions including Na^+, K^+ coupled with the movement of Cl^- and water into the cell can lead to extracellular space (ECS) shrinkage, further contributing to neuronal excitability [42]. Inhibition of changes in ECS volume to reduce cerebral edema may be a potential target in treating patients with refractory epilepsies including PTE [43].

Cell swelling can occur during seizures, and glial swelling may promote pathological neuronal firing while neuronal swelling may have protective effects. Following neuronal depolarization, extracellular K^+ is taken up by perisynaptic astrocytes mainly through Kir4.1. One hypothesis is that Kir4.1 channels may indirectly facilitate water uptake into astrocytes through the astrocyte water channel aquaporin-4 (AQP4), which could promote increased excitability through a reduction in extracellular space volume [44–46].

Tight junctions and posttraumatic epilepsy

Tight junctions between neighboring brain capillary endothelial cells maintain BBB integrity while astrocytic endfeet regulate endothelial blood flux [47,48]. Disruption of tight junction complexes following TBI results in increased paracellular permeability promoting influx of inflammatory cells, blood-borne proteins, and albumin which can lead to a cascade of events ultimately influencing neuronal and glial function [49] (Fig. 9.6). Matrix metalloproteinases (MMPs) regulate the extracellular matrix (ECM) and could affect BBB integrity following injury through digestion and remodeling of the ECM surrounding brain capillaries and degradation of tight junction proteins [50,51]. MMP-2 and MMP-9 modulate tight junction integrity, and elevation of MMP-9 increases acutely after TBI and has been shown to promote epileptogenesis after TBI [52–54]. Transgenic mice that overexpress MMP-9 have an increased susceptibility to developing spontaneous seizures following CCI, while MMP-9 knockout mice have decreased epileptiform activity 3.5 months following CCI-induced TBI [53]. Latency to first epileptiform discharge following injection of the convulsant pentylenetetrazole (PTZ) in CCI-injured animals is also decreased in mice overexpressing MMP-9 and increased in MMP-9 knockout mice, suggesting a correlation between MMP-9 genotype and PTZ-induced seizure susceptibility [53]. MMP-9 levels are also increased in patients following TBI [55], and serum MMP levels are correlated to

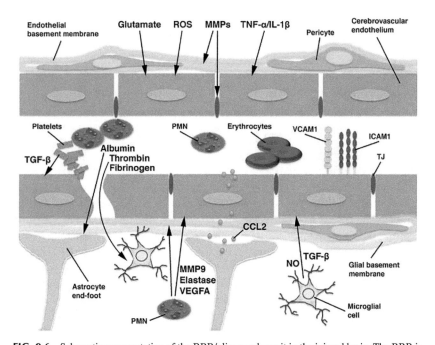

FIG. 9.6   Schematic representation of the BBB/gliovascular unit in the injured brain. The BBB is formed by the brain endothelial cells connected by tight junctions (TJs). However, astrocytes, whose end feet make an intimate contact with the cerebrovascular endothelium, are critical for normal function of the BBB. Microglial processes are also closely associated with the brain endothelium in 4%–13% of cerebral microvessels, and glial and endothelial cells functionally interact with each other in a paracrine manner. Brain parenchymal cells are normally shielded from periphery by the BBB. However, the disruption of vascular integrity occurring after neurotrauma allows blood-borne factors, such as albumin and fibrinogen, as well as thrombin, which is cleaved from prothrombin by Factor Xa, to enter the brain. Fibrinogen, after its conversion to fibrin, acts on microglia, causing the rearrangement of microglial cytoskeleton and increased phagocytosis. Thrombin predominantly acts on microglia, stimulating their proliferation and inducing the production of nitric oxide (NO). It also increases the microglial synthesis of proinflammatory mediators, such as tumor necrosis factor-α (TNF-α) and interleukin (IL)-6 and -12. In addition, thrombin may target the cerebrovascular endothelium and increase the permeability of the BBB. Similar to thrombin, albumin promotes the proliferation of microglial cells and increases the production of NO and proinflammatory mediators, such as IL-1β. Albumin also acts on astrocytes by binding to transforming growth factor-β (TGF-β) receptor II, which may play a role in posttraumatic cortical epileptogenesis. Among the putative factors contributing to posttraumatic dysfunction of the BBB are glutamate, reactive oxygen species (ROS), matrix metalloproteinases (MMPs), proinflammatory cytokines TNF-α and IL-1β, and vascular endothelial growth factor A (VEGFA). After injury, glutamate is released from various parenchymal cells and from invading neutrophils (polymorphonuclear leukocytes, PMN). It increases the permeability of the BBB and has been shown to promote apoptosis of brain endothelial cells, although this latter action of glutamate has been questioned. ROS not only increase the permeability of brain endothelium, but also play an important role in promoting posttraumatic invasion of inflammatory cells by upregulating the endothelial expression of cell adhesion molecules, such as intercellular adhesion molecule-1 (ICAM1). MMPs are produced by multiple types of parenchymal cells and can also be released from invading leukocytes. MMPs disrupt the integrity of the BBB by attacking basal lamina proteins and degrading tight junctions. TNF-α and IL-1β increase the

BBB dysfunction following TBI. Serum MMP-7 levels are positively correlated with BBB dysfunction, measuring K^{Trans} ratios, using dynamic contrast-enhanced MRI (DCE-MRI) [56]. A peripheral biomarker, such as serum MMP levels, that is correlated with a validated radiological measure of BBB dysfunction, could assist in serial assessment of BBB dysfunction and patient treatment. The MMP-2/9 inhibitor IPR-179 has been shown to have antiseizure and antiepileptic effects in the intrahippocampal kainic acid model of epilepsy [57]. Specifically, rats treated with IPR-179 starting 24 h after kainic acid injection have significantly lower seizure frequencies and seizure durations compared to vehicle-treated rats [57]. These data suggest that MMP inhibition could be a promising prophylactic treatment for PTE, and should be further investigated.

Glial influence on the blood-brain barrier and posttraumatic epilepsy

Aquaporins

The aquaporins (AQPs) are a family of membrane proteins that function as water channels facilitating the transport of water to and from cells through osmotic gradients [58,59]. AQP4 is the main water channel expressed in the CNS and is predominantly found on astrocytic endfeet found at the border between the brain parenchyma and the major fluid compartments: the CSF and blood [60,61]. AQP4 knockout (KO) mice display markedly prolonged stimulation-induced seizures and slowed potassium kinetics in comparison with wild-type (WT) mice [62]. Following TBI, AQP4 KO mice have increased spontaneous seizure duration compared to control mice, suggesting that AQP4 might play a role in seizure termination as well [63]. In mice that develop PTE following CCI, AQP4

FIG. 9.6, CONT'D   permeability of the BBB, but, more importantly, they also play a key role in progression of posttraumatic neuroinflammation. These cytokines increase the endothelial expression of cell adhesion molecules, such as *E*-selectin, ICAM1, and vascular cell adhesion molecule-1 (VCAM1). They also induce the endothelial and astrocytic production of CXC and CC chemokines, including CXCL1, -2, and CCL2, which attract circulating inflammatory cells and facilitate their migration across the BBB. Astrocyte-derived CCL2 can be transported across the cerebrovascular endothelium and then presented on its luminal surface. This chemokine can also increase the permeability of the BBB. VEGFA increases the permeability of brain endothelium by changing the distribution and downregulating the expression of tight junction proteins. After injury, VEGFA is predominantly produced by astrocytes, but is also carried by invading neutrophils. The major source of TGF-β is the aggregating platelets, but TGF-β is also produced by microglia and, to a lesser extent, by astrocytes. TGF-β has been shown to increase the permeability of the cerebrovascular endothelium; however, other investigators postulated that this growth factor has an opposite effect on the BBB, which is to enhance and maintain the barrier properties of brain endothelium. Invading neutrophils exert an adverse effect on BBB function. These inflammatory cells not only produce proinflammatory cytokines, such as TNF-α, and generate large amounts of ROS, but they also release various proteolytic enzymes, including MMP-9 and neutrophil elastase. *(Reproduced with permission from Chodobski A, et al. Blood-brain barrier pathophysiology in traumatic brain injury. Transl Stroke Res 2011;2(4):492–516.)*

is also mislocalized away from the perivascular endfeet and toward the neuropil which could lead to impaired water and ion homeostasis [24]. Upregulation of AQP4 has been shown to improve BBB integrity and edema following intracerebral hemorrhage, suggesting that AQP4 enhancers could be used as a BBB-modulating target to alleviate the edema that occurs following traumatic injury [64]. Alternatively, inhibiting AQP4 expression using small-interfering RNA (siRNA) after CCI in rats decreases BBB disruption, reduces astrogliosis, increases microglial activation in the perilesional cortex, and increases neuronal survival in the hippocampus [65]. Clinical agent AER-271, a selective AQP4 antagonist, recently underwent a double-blind placebo-controlled phase 1 study with results pending (NCT03804476). These dissimilar findings suggest that further investigation into the role of AQP4 in PTE is essential to determine whether AQP4 regulation is neuroprotective or exacerbates disease following injury. These conflicting results may be due to the divergent roles these channels play in edema generation and clearance at different phases of epileptogenesis [66].

Cation-chloride cotransporters

Na^+-K^+-Cl^- cotransporter (NKCC1) and K^+-Cl^- cotransporter (KCC2) are the two main cation-chloride cotransporters (CCCs) that have been shown to play a role in the development of epilepsy. NKCC1, which is expressed in neurons and glial cells throughout the brain, brings Cl^- into neurons pushing gamma-aminobutyric acid (GABA) into a more depolarizing function [67]. In contrast, KCC2 is expressed in the plasma membrane of somata and dendrites of pyramidal neurons and interneurons in the hippocampus and neocortex, and it functions to bring Cl^- out of the cell and therefore has the opposite effect [68,69]. These transporters work to regulate the concentrations of Na^+, K^+, and Cl^- based on their respective electrochemical gradients.

In the adult brain, NKCC1 activity is downregulated while KCC2 activity is upregulated resulting in Cl^- extrusion to become more dominant in the adult brain switching GABA to become hyperpolarizing. Dysregulation of these transporters can promote a switch to depolarizing GABA and ictogenesis [42,70]. Blocking KCC2 activity promotes status epilepticus-like events in tissue [71]. Conversely, the NKCC1 blocker bumetanide has been shown to have promising antiseizure effects across multiple studies [72–75].

Serum albumin and astrocytic transforming growth factor-beta signaling

BBB leakage exposes the brain to albumin, and albumin can be taken up by astrocytes. Albumin uptake by astrocytes is mediated by TGF-β receptors and leads to activation of astrocytes and decreased capacity to buffer extracellular K^+, which can in turn increase neuronal excitability and epileptiform activity [16]. Serum-derived albumin induces activation of the activin-receptor-like kinase 5 (ALK5) pathway of TGF-β receptor 1 in astrocytes following injury and can also upregulate the expression of TGF-β receptors in a positive feedback loop [76]. Blocking TGF-β receptors reduces the amount of albumin taken up by astrocytes and prevents albumin-induced epilepsy [16,76]. In a rat model of vascular injury and BBB breakdown, losartan, an FDA-approved drug known to block TGF-β signaling, reduces the percentage of animals that develop postinjury epilepsy and reduce the number of seizures in animals that develop epilepsy [76]. Blocking TGF-β signaling using losartan prevents albumin-induced epilepsy and therefore could be antiepileptic in patients with TBI-associated vascular injuries [76,77] (Fig. 9.7). The astrocytic ALK5/TGF-β pathway that is activated by the presence of serum albumin in the extracellular space induces excitatory but not inhibitory synaptogenesis preceding the appearance of seizures, suggesting that albumin can selectively induce epileptogenesis through glutamatergic transmission [78] (Fig. 9.8). Altogether, these data indicate that the ALK5/TGF-β pathway could be a promising therapeutic target in the early prevention of PTE.

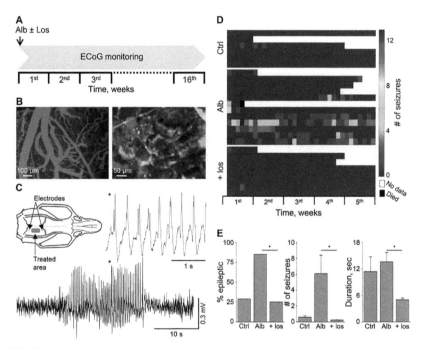

FIG. 9.7 Losartan prevents albumin-induced epilepsy. (A) Treatment protocol; animals were treated with local application of albumin (Alb) in the presence or absence of losartan (Los), added to the artificial cerebrospinal fluid (ACSF). (B) *In vivo* imaging of cortical vessels during local application of fluorescently labeled albumin *(green)* and Evans blue (EB, *red*) intravenous injection, indicating no EB extravasation, consistent with normally functioning BBB. (C) The development of epilepsy was assessed through the occurrence of spontaneous electrocorticographic seizures (see exemplary seizure of an albumin-treated rat). (D) Color-coded table showing the number of seizures per day is presented for each rat in albumin (Alb)- compared to ACSF (Ctrl)- and losartan (Los)-treated animals (see scale bar). (E) Bar graphs represent the percent of epileptic animals, number of seizures per week, and the duration of seizures. Overall, compared to the albumin group, losartan treatment significantly lowered the percent of epileptic animals, and the number and duration of seizures among animals that did develop epilepsy. *$P \leq .05$. *(Reproduced with permission from Bar-Klein G, et al. Losartan prevents acquired epilepsy via TGF-beta signaling suppression. Ann Neurol 2014;75(6):864–75.)*

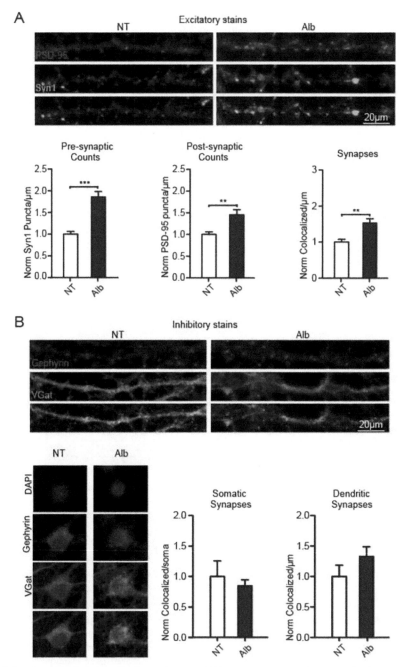

FIG. 9.8 Albumin induces excitatory, but not inhibitory, synaptogenesis in temporal cultures. (A) Staining for excitatory presynaptic (Syn1; *green*) and postsynaptic (PSD-95, *red*) proteins, revealed a significant albumin-induced increase in presynaptic, postsynaptic, and colocalized counts along dendritic lengths (Alb=17; no treatment (NT)=12). (B) Staining for inhibitory presynaptic (V-Gat, *green*) and postsynaptic (gephyrin, *red*) proteins showed no significant albumin-induced differences in synaptic counts, quantified along dendritic lengths and the somatic area (per soma: Alb=17; NT=15; P=.2569; and per dendrite Alb=19; NT=18. P=.0854). Error bars indicate SEM. *P ≤ .05, **P ≤ .01, ***P ≤ .001. *(Reproduced with permission from Weissberg I, et al. Albumin induces excitatory synaptogenesis through astrocytic TGF-beta/ALK5 signaling in a model of acquired epilepsy following blood-brain barrier dysfunction. Neurobiol Dis 2015;78:115–25.)*

Chronic BBB disruption and the downstream molecular changes it effects play an important role in the pathogenesis of PTE. Lasting BBB pathology is a common finding across animal models and in patients with PTE. Following TBI, BBB permeability is increased in patients that develop PTE compared to patients without epilepsy. In patients, BBB integrity can be evaluated noninvasively with MRI, and this could be a valuable tool to predict risk for developing epilepsy following TBI. Disrupting the BBB in animals leads to epileptogenesis, potentially through albumin-induced excitatory synaptogenesis and activation of astrocytes. Activated astrocytes in animal models of PTE display mislocalization of AQP4 while inhibition of AQP4 has been shown to improve BBB integrity and neuronal survival, suggesting a potential target for the prevention of PTE. Taken together, the BBB is a dynamic structure and disruption of its integrity could contribute to the development of PTE following TBI.

References

[1] Daneman R, Prat A. The blood-brain barrier. Cold Spring Harb Perspect Biol 2015;7(1), a020412.

[2] Gennarelli T, Graham D. Textbook of traumatic brain injury. Washington, DC: American Psychiatric Publishing, Inc.; 2005. p. 27–50.

[3] Liddelow SA. Fluids and barriers of the CNS: a historical viewpoint. Fluids Barriers CNS 2011;8(1):2.

[4] Goldmann EE. Die äussere und innere Sekretion des gesunden und kranken Organismus im Lichte der 'vitalen Färbung'. Beitr Klin Chir 1909;64:192–265.

[5] Goldmann EE. Vitalfärbung am Zentralnervensystem. In: Abhandlungen Preussischen Akademie der Wissenschaften Physikalisch Mathematisch klasse, vol. I; 1913. p. 1–60.

[6] Jiang JY, et al. Moderate hypothermia reduces blood-brain barrier disruption following traumatic brain injury in the rat. Acta Neuropathol 1992;84(5):495–500.

[7] Dietrich WD, Alonso O, Halley M. Early microvascular and neuronal consequences of traumatic brain injury: a light and electron microscopic study in rats. J Neurotrauma 1994;11(3):289–301.

[8] Mikawa S, et al. Attenuation of acute and chronic damage following traumatic brain injury in copper, zinc-superoxide dismutase transgenic mice. J Neurosurg 1996;85(5):885–91.

[9] Hartl R, et al. Blood-brain barrier breakdown occurs early after traumatic brain injury and is not related to white blood cell adherence. Acta Neurochir Suppl 1997;70:240–2.

[10] Adelson PD, et al. Blood brain barrier permeability and acute inflammation in two models of traumatic brain injury in the immature rat: a preliminary report. Acta Neurochir Suppl 1998;71:104–6.

[11] Lammie GA, et al. Neuropathologic characterization of a rodent model of closed head injury—addition of clinically relevant secondary insults does not significantly potentiate brain damage. J Neurotrauma 1999;16(7):603–15.

[12] Shlosberg D, et al. Blood-brain barrier breakdown as a therapeutic target in traumatic brain injury. Nat Rev Neurol 2010;6(7):393–403.

[13] van Vliet EA, et al. Long-lasting blood-brain barrier dysfunction and neuroinflammation after traumatic brain injury. Neurobiol Dis 2020;145, 105080.

[14] van Vliet EA, et al. Longitudinal assessment of blood-brain barrier leakage during epileptogenesis in rats. A quantitative MRI study. Neurobiol Dis 2014;63:74–84.

[15] Seiffert E, et al. Lasting blood-brain barrier disruption induces epileptic focus in the rat somatosensory cortex. J Neurosci 2004;24(36):7829–36.

[16] Ivens S, et al. TGF-beta receptor-mediated albumin uptake into astrocytes is involved in neocortical epileptogenesis. Brain 2007;130(Pt 2):535–47.

[17] Tomkins O, et al. Blood-brain barrier disruption results in delayed functional and structural alterations in the rat neocortex. Neurobiol Dis 2007;25(2):367–77.

[18] Kim SY, et al. TGFbeta signaling is associated with changes in inflammatory gene expression and perineuronal net degradation around inhibitory neurons following various neurological insults. Sci Rep 2017;7(1):7711.

[19] D'Ambrosio R, et al. Impaired K(+) homeostasis and altered electrophysiological properties of post-traumatic hippocampal glia. J Neurosci 1999;19(18):8152–62.

[20] Stewart TH, et al. Chronic dysfunction of astrocytic inwardly rectifying K+ channels specific to the neocortical epileptic focus after fluid percussion injury in the rat. J Neurophysiol 2010;104(6):3345–60.

[21] Takahashi H, Manaka S, Sano K. Changes in extracellular potassium concentration in cortex and brain stem during the acute phase of experimental closed head injury. J Neurosurg 1981;55(5):708–17.

[22] Katayama Y, et al. Massive increases in extracellular potassium and the indiscriminate release of glutamate following concussive brain injury. J Neurosurg 1990;73(6):889–900.

[23] Santhakumar V, et al. Post-traumatic hyperexcitability is not caused by impaired buffering of extracellular potassium. J Neurosci 2003;23(13):5865–76.

[24] Szu JI, et al. Aquaporin-4 dysregulation in a controlled cortical impact injury model of posttraumatic epilepsy. Neuroscience 2020;428:140–53.

[25] Reiber H, Felgenhauer K. Protein transfer at the blood cerebrospinal fluid barrier and the quantitation of the humoral immune response within the central nervous system. Clin Chim Acta 1987;163(3):319–28.

[26] Tibbling G, Link H, Ohman S. Principles of albumin and IgG analyses in neurological disorders. I. Establishment of reference values. Scand J Clin Lab Invest 1977;37(5):385–90.

[27] Yan EB, et al. Post-traumatic hypoxia is associated with prolonged cerebral cytokine production, higher serum biomarker levels, and poor outcome in patients with severe traumatic brain injury. J Neurotrauma 2014;31(7):618–29.

[28] Correale J, et al. Status epilepticus increases CSF levels of neuron-specific enolase and alters the blood-brain barrier. Neurology 1998;50(5):1388–91.

[29] Tomkins O, et al. Blood-brain barrier disruption in post-traumatic epilepsy. J Neurol Neurosurg Psychiatry 2008;79(7):774–7.

[30] Tomkins O, et al. Blood-brain barrier breakdown following traumatic brain injury: a possible role in posttraumatic epilepsy. Cardiovasc Psychiatry Neurol 2011;2011, 765923.

[31] Hoffman SN, Salin PA, Prince DA. Chronic neocortical epileptogenesis in vitro. J Neurophysiol 1994;71(5):1762–73.

[32] Fabene PF, et al. A role for leukocyte-endothelial adhesion mechanisms in epilepsy. Nat Med 2008;14(12):1377–83.

[33] Janigro D. Are you in or out? Leukocyte, ion, and neurotransmitter permeability across the epileptic blood-brain barrier. Epilepsia 2012;53(Suppl 1):26–34.

[34] Pavlovsky L, et al. Persistent BBB disruption may underlie alpha interferon-induced seizures. J Neurol 2005;252(1):42–6.

[35] Janssen HL, et al. Seizures associated with low-dose alpha-interferon. Lancet 1990;336(8730):1580.

[36] Woynarowski M, Socha J. Seizures in children during interferon alpha therapy. J Hepatol 1997;26(4):956–7.

[37] Unterberg AW, et al. Edema and brain trauma. Neuroscience 2004;129(4):1021–9.

[38] Donkin JJ, Vink R. Mechanisms of cerebral edema in traumatic brain injury: therapeutic developments. Curr Opin Neurol 2010;23(3):293–9.

[39] Stokum JA, Gerzanich V, Simard JM. Molecular pathophysiology of cerebral edema. J Cereb Blood Flow Metab 2016;36(3):513–38.

[40] Michinaga S, Koyama Y. Pathogenesis of brain edema and investigation into anti-edema drugs. Int J Mol Sci 2015;16(5):9949–75.

[41] Nehring SM, Tadi P, Tenny S. Cerebral edema. Treasure Island, FL: StatPearls; 2021.

[42] Colbourn R, Naik A, Hrabetova S. ECS dynamism and its influence on neuronal excitability and seizures. Neurochem Res 2019;44(5):1020–36.

[43] Colbourn R, et al. Rapid volume pulsation of the extracellular space coincides with epileptiform activity in mice and depends on the NBCe1 transporter. J Physiol 2021;599(12):3195–220.

[44] Murphy TR, Binder DK, Fiacco TA. Turning down the volume: astrocyte volume change in the generation and termination of epileptic seizures. Neurobiol Dis 2017;104:24–32.

[45] Kinboshi M, Ikeda A, Ohno Y. Role of astrocytic inwardly rectifying potassium (Kir) 4.1 channels in epileptogenesis. Front Neurol 2020;11, 626658.

[46] Hibino H, et al. Inwardly rectifying potassium channels: their structure, function, and physiological roles. Physiol Rev 2010;90(1):291–366.

[47] Abbott NJ, et al. Structure and function of the blood-brain barrier. Neurobiol Dis 2010;37(1):13–25.

[48] Alvarez JI, Katayama T, Prat A. Glial influence on the blood brain barrier. Glia 2013;61(12):1939–58.

[49] Chodobski A, Zink BJ, Szmydynger-Chodobska J. Blood-brain barrier pathophysiology in traumatic brain injury. Transl Stroke Res 2011;2(4):492–516.

[50] Lischper M, et al. Metalloproteinase mediated occludin cleavage in the cerebral microcapillary endothelium under pathological conditions. Brain Res 2010;1326:114–27.

[51] Mun-Bryce S, Rosenberg GA. Gelatinase B modulates selective opening of the blood-brain barrier during inflammation. Am J Physiol 1998;274(5):R1203–11.

[52] Vermeer PD, et al. MMP9 modulates tight junction integrity and cell viability in human airway epithelia. Am J Physiol Lung Cell Mol Physiol 2009;296(5):L751–62.

[53] Pijet B, et al. Elevation of MMP-9 levels promotes epileptogenesis after traumatic brain injury. Mol Neurobiol 2018;55(12):9294–306.

[54] Feng S, et al. Matrix metalloproteinase-2 and -9 secreted by leukemic cells increase the permeability of blood-brain barrier by disrupting tight junction proteins. PLoS One 2011;6(8), e20599.

[55] Suehiro E, et al. Increased matrix metalloproteinase-9 in blood in association with activation of interleukin-6 after traumatic brain injury: influence of hypothermic therapy. J Neurotrauma 2004;21(12):1706–11.

[56] Nichols P, et al. Blood-brain barrier dysfunction significantly correlates with serum matrix metalloproteinase-7 (MMP-7) following traumatic brain injury. Neuroimage Clin 2021;31, 102741.

[57] Broekaart DW, et al. The matrix metalloproteinase inhibitor IPR-179 has antiseizure and antiepileptogenic effects. J Clin Invest 2021;131(1).

[58] Verkman AS. Physiological importance of aquaporin water channels. Ann Med 2002;34(3):192–200.

[59] Verkman AS. More than just water channels: unexpected cellular roles of aquaporins. J Cell Sci 2005;118(Pt 15):3225–32.

[60] Nielsen S, et al. Specialized membrane domains for water transport in glial cells: high-resolution immunogold cytochemistry of aquaporin-4 in rat brain. J Neurosci 1997;17(1):171–80.

[61] Nagelhus EA, Mathiisen TM, Ottersen OP. Aquaporin-4 in the central nervous system: cellular and subcellular distribution and coexpression with KIR4.1. Neuroscience 2004;129(4):905–13.

[62] Binder DK, et al. Increased seizure duration and slowed potassium kinetics in mice lacking aquaporin-4 water channels. Glia 2006;53(6):631–6.

[63] Szu JI, et al. Modulation of posttraumatic epileptogenesis in aquaporin-4 knockout mice. Epilepsia 2020;61(7):1503–14.

[64] Jeon H, et al. Upregulation of AQP4 improves blood-brain barrier integrity and perihematomal edema following intracerebral hemorrhage. Neurotherapeutics 2021;18(4):2692–706.

[65] Fukuda AM, et al. Posttraumatic reduction of edema with aquaporin-4 RNA interference improves acute and chronic functional recovery. J Cereb Blood Flow Metab 2013;33(10):1621–32.

[66] Jha RM, et al. Emerging therapeutic targets for cerebral edema. Expert Opin Ther Targets 2021;25(11):917–38.

[67] Yamada J, et al. Cl- uptake promoting depolarizing GABA actions in immature rat neocortical neurons is mediated by NKCC1. J Physiol 2004;557(Pt 3):829–41.

[68] Chamma I, et al. Role of the neuronal K-cl co-transporter KCC2 in inhibitory and excitatory neurotransmission. Front Cell Neurosci 2012;6:5.

[69] Kaila K, et al. Cation-chloride cotransporters in neuronal development, plasticity and disease. Nat Rev Neurosci 2014;15(10):637–54.

[70] Liu R, et al. Role of NKCC1 and KCC2 in epilepsy: from expression to function. Front Neurol 2019;10:1407.

[71] Gonzalez MI. Regulation of the cell surface expression of chloride transporters during epileptogenesis. Neurosci Lett 2016;628:213–8.

[72] Dzhala V, Staley KJ. Acute and chronic efficacy of bumetanide in an in vitro model of posttraumatic epileptogenesis. CNS Neurosci Ther 2015;21(2):173–80.

[73] Mazarati A, Shin D, Sankar R. Bumetanide inhibits rapid kindling in neonatal rats. Epilepsia 2009;50(9):2117–22.

[74] Edwards DA, et al. Bumetanide alleviates epileptogenic and neurotoxic effects of sevoflurane in neonatal rat brain. Anesthesiology 2010;112(3):567–75.

[75] Sivakumaran S, Maguire J. Bumetanide reduces seizure progression and the development of pharmacoresistant status epilepticus. Epilepsia 2016;57(2):222–32.

[76] Bar-Klein G, et al. Losartan prevents acquired epilepsy via TGF-beta signaling suppression. Ann Neurol 2014;75(6):864–75.

[77] Friedman A, et al. Should losartan be administered following brain injury? Expert Rev Neurother 2014;14(12):1365–75.

[78] Weissberg I, et al. Albumin induces excitatory synaptogenesis through astrocytic TGF-beta/ALK5 signaling in a model of acquired epilepsy following blood-brain barrier dysfunction. Neurobiol Dis 2015;78:115–25.

Chapter 10

Inflammation and posttraumatic epilepsy

Overview

Following traumatic brain injury (TBI), a neuroinflammatory response is initiated that leads to the release of cytokines, chemokines, and the infiltration of peripheral immune cells. Astrocytes and resident microglia are activated which leads to migration and proliferation at the site of injury. Both acute and chronic neuroinflammation following TBI may contribute to the development of epilepsy. In healthy tissue, inflammation plays an important role in combating pathogens and restoring tissue homeostasis, but prolonged inflammation observed following TBI can exacerbate tissue damage. Studies support a pro-epileptogenic role of neuroinflammation following TBI which suggests that inhibition of these pathways could be therapeutically targeted in posttraumatic epilepsy (PTE). In this chapter, we will discuss the current understanding of how inflammation may contribute to the development of PTE and whether inflammatory mediators could be used to identify risk factors for the development of PTE.

Chronic neuroinflammation and seizure susceptibility

Neuroinflammation can be observed months to years following TBI in patients and animal models and may contribute to the development of epilepsy [1–4] (Fig. 10.1). The main features of the inflammatory response in the brain following injury include microglial and astrocytic activation and migration, release of inflammatory factors, and recruitment of blood-derived leukocytes into the brain. Following TBI, there is an increase in many pro-inflammatory mediators in the brain including tumor necrosis factor-alpha (TNF-α), interleukins, and migration inhibitory factor (MIF) which have been implicated in the development of epilepsy following injury [1,5] (Fig. 10.2).

Posttraumatic Epilepsy. https://doi.org/10.1016/B978-0-323-90099-7.00012-5

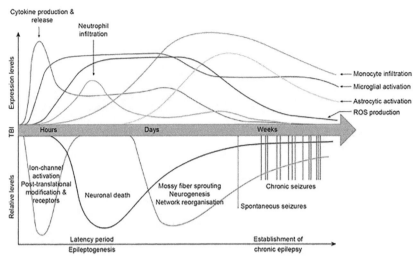

FIG. 10.1 Summary of the progression of inflammatory factors and epileptogenesis after TBI. After TBI, epileptogenesis occurs after a latent period of months to years. Within hours after the injury, a myriad of cytokines are released at high levels which can continue for days. This is concurrent with activation of ion channels and posttranslational modifications of various receptors associated with neuronal excitation and inhibition, which can occur as early as minutes after the injury. Local immune cells are activated, and peripheral immune cells are also recruited to the area within hours to days. Neuroinflammation can persist for weeks after the injury, coincident with widespread neuronal loss. In the later phase of epileptogenesis, processes such as neurogenesis and mossy fiber sprouting in the hippocampus contribute to an increasingly excitable neuronal environment. It may be weeks, months, or years before spontaneous seizures and the establishment of chronic and persistent epilepsy manifests. *(Reproduced with permission from Webster KM, et al. Inflammation in epileptogenesis after traumatic brain injury. J Neuroinflammation 2017;14(1):10.)*

Glial cells

Activated microglia

Microglia, the resident innate immune cells of the central nervous system (CNS), perform primary immune surveillance and macrophage-like activities, including production and release of cytokines and chemokines [6]. Chronic microglial activation can be observed months to years following injury in patients and animal models [2,3]. CD68-positive cells, a marker for activated macrophages/monocytes/microglia, can be observed in the lesion core and perilesional area 11 months following fluid percussion injury (FPI) in rats [3]. In addition, CD68-positive cells can be observed in the ipsilateral thalamus and in the dentate gyrus of the ipsilateral hippocampus 11 months postinjury in these rats [3]. These data suggest that chronic inflammation can be observed not only in the perilesional zone but also at distant sites following brain injury [3]. Interestingly, this group did not find an association between increased perilesional neuroinflammation and seizure susceptibility. In fact, CD68 immunoreactivity in the perilesional cortex is greater in rats with no increase in seizure susceptibility as compared to

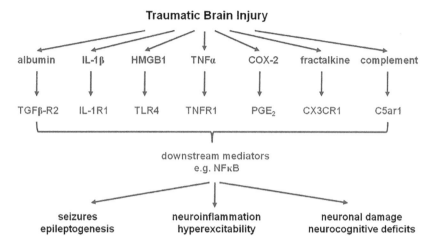

FIG. 10.2 TBI triggers the upregulation of a wide range of pro-inflammatory mediators and their signaling pathways. Many of these, including those noted here, have been implicated in the development of epilepsy based on observations in patient samples as well as experimental manipulations in small animal models. Abbreviations: COX-2, cyclooxygenase-2; CX3CR1, CX3C chemokine receptor 1; C5ar1, complement component 5a receptor 1; HMGB1, high mobility group box protein 1; IL-1β, interleukin-1 beta; IL-1R1, interleukin-1 receptor 1; NFκB, nuclear factor kappa-B; PGE2, prostaglandin E2; MAPK, p38 mitogen activated protein kinase; TGF-β, transforming growth factor-beta; TLR4, Toll-like receptor 4; TNF-α, tumor necrosis factor-alpha; TNFR1, tumor necrosis factor receptor 1. *(Reproduced with permission from Saletti PG, et al. In search of antiepileptogenic treatments for posttraumatic epilepsy. Neurobiol Dis 2019;123:86–99.)*

those with increased seizure susceptibility when challenged with the convulsant pentylenetetrazole (PTZ).

Microglial activation following TBI can be heterogeneous, driving both pro- and anti-inflammatory phenotypes. Following TBI, microglia typically display both M1 and M2 activation in the acute phase, while the injury site is dominated by the M1-like phenotype at chronic time points which may contribute to increased cortical and hippocampal neuronal death [7]. Microglia can undergo classical activation, M1-like phenotype, which is pro-inflammatory and regulates clearance of cell debris following injury, but chronic M1 polarization could result in damage to the brain. M1-like activated microglia can release pro-inflammatory mediators including interleukin-1 beta (IL-1β), TNF-α, and high-mobility group box 1 (HMGB1) which may contribute to epileptogenesis [4,8,9].

HMGB1, a DNA-binding protein, has been shown to play a key role in neuroinflammation following TBI and epilepsy. Elevated cerebrospinal fluid (CSF) and serum levels of HMGB1 have been observed in patients with epilepsy [10,11]. Serum HMGB1 levels are also higher in patients with an average seizure duration >5 min compared to patients with a seizure duration <5 min, suggesting that HMGB1 levels could potentially be used to predict risk and severity of epilepsy [10]. Inhibition of HMGB1 with glycyrrhizin following injury reduces chronic microglial reactivity, calculated as ionized calcium-binding adaptor molecule 1 (Iba1) relative intensity, in the hippocampus 6 months following controlled cortical impact (CCI) injury in young mice [12]. Interestingly, there is no difference in Iba1 reactivity in the cortex lesion core of glycyrrhizin-treated mice compared to sham mice. Although inhibition of HMGB1 with glycyrrhizin prevents spatial and motor deficits, it does not affect seizure duration in mice that develop chronic spontaneous seizures. In the above study, 5 months following TBI, 15% of mice treated with vehicle developed spontaneous seizures while 7% of mice treated with glycyrrhizin developed seizures, but the proportion of epileptic animals did not differ significantly between groups possibly due to the low yield of mice developing PTE [12]. These data suggest that inhibition of HMGB1 could have antiepileptic effects following TBI, but further studies are needed to explore this. These data also bring to light the importance of developing better preclinical PTE models suitable for biomarker discovery and drug testing [13] (Chapters 6 and 7).

Microglia can also undergo alternative activation, the M2-like phenotype, and release anti-inflammatory mediators that promote repair mechanisms. M2-like microglia downregulate M1 signaling by releasing anti-inflammatory cytokines like interleukin-10 (IL-10) and interleukin-13 (IL-13). M2-like microglia can also release growth factors that support regeneration including transforming growth factor-beta (TGF-β) and insulin-like growth factor 1 [14]. M2-like response becomes suppressed over time following CCI in mice which could polarize microglia to a pro-inflammatory state [7]. Mixed microglia polarization is observed prior to seizure onset, but M1-like phenotype dominates acutely before the onset of spontaneous seizures [15]. These data suggest that microglial polarization could potentially be used as a biomarker in predicting the development of epilepsy following TBI, and driving M2-like polarization in macrophages could possibly be used as a strategy to prevent PTE [16].

Astrogliosis

Astrogliosis and astrocyte hypertrophy may contribute to aberrant neurogenesis and hyperexcitability following TBI. Radial glial-like processes that extend through the granule cell layer of the hippocampus were reduced whereas glial fibrillary acidic protein positive (GFAP+) cells displayed hypertrophied processes at the base of the granule cell layer 30 days following FPI compared to sham mice [17]. This group also observed that basal dendrites from the doublecortin-positive (DCX+) cells, a marker for immature neurons, extended deep into the hilus in mice 30 days after FPI. Dendritic abnormalities have the potential to create new pathways for excitatory circuitry in the hippocampus [18]. Interestingly, these mice also had an increase in the number of immature granule cells in the hilus compared to sham mice. These data suggest that astrocyte hypertrophy may contribute to aberrant sprouting of basal dendrites which could contribute to epileptogenesis following TBI [17,19].

Interestingly, astrocytes have been shown to respond differently to various types of TBI. In a model of repetitive diffuse closed-head TBI (rdTBI) that induces only diffuse injury, astrocytes do not form glial scars and upregulation of GFAP is limited [20]. Using a marker for the cell cycle, the protein Ki67, this group also determined that rdTBI did not induce proliferation of GFAP + astrocytes which is a common finding following brain injury. Interestingly, in a subset of astrocytes, glutamate transporter-1 (GLT-1), glutamine synthetase (GS), and the inwardly rectifying potassium channel Kir4.1 were downregulated in the cortical gray matter of mice following injury [20]. This group observed a decrease in GLT-1 expression, which appeared as patches of GLT-1 loss, in these "atypical" astrocytes up to 3 months following injury. Interestingly, these "atypical" astrocytes were uncoupled from other astrocytes in these mice. Furthermore, mice that developed PTE had significantly greater GLT-1 area loss compared to mice that did not develop PTE following rdTBI (Fig. 10.3).

Cytokines

Cytokines produced following TBI may be associated with the development of PTE. Cytokines shown to be dysregulated following injury that could contribute to seizures include interleukins, TNF-α, HMGB1, and MIF [12,21–23]. IL-1β, HMGB1, and MIF have been shown to have a more pro-inflammatory response promoting hyperexcitability while IL-10 has been shown to have antiseizure effects. Alternatively, TNF-α has been shown to have heterogeneous effects in different models [24–26].

Interleukin-1 beta

IL-1β is a pro-inflammatory cytokine that is produced by microglia and astrocytes in the CNS. IL-1β has been shown to increase neuronal excitability through calcium, glutamatergic, and GABAergic mechanisms which could contribute to the development of epilepsy [27]. Following TBI, higher CSF/serum IL-1β ratios in patients during the first week postinjury are associated with increased risk for PTE over time [28]. Studies have identified multiple single-nucleotide polymorphisms (SNPs) associated with increased seizure risk following brain injury [29,30]. Patients with the rs1143634 SNP in the IL-1β gene show an increased risk for PTE compared to patients with alternative genotypes. Patients that were heterozygous at RS1143634 have an increased risk of PTE and had significantly shorter time to first seizure (5 months shorter on average) compared to homozygotes [28]. This group suggests that heterozygote associations for genetic variation could lead to a mixture of IL-1β isoforms with downstream signaling within inflammatory pathways that could lead to increased risk for PTE. In principle, genetic profiling of patients to examine these risk alleles following TBI could help determine the best medication for that individual to prevent or reduce the risk of PTE.

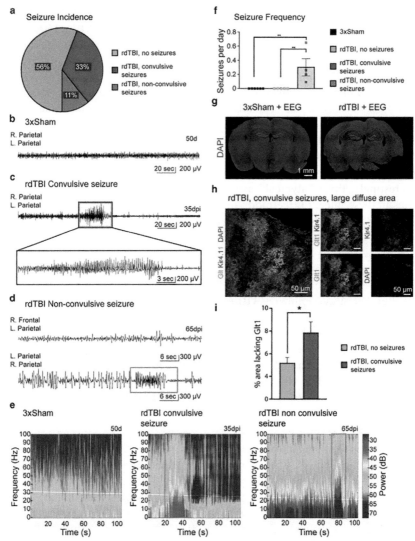

FIG. 10.3 rdTBI causes spontaneous, unprovoked, recurrent seizures. (A) Pie chart representing the incidence of seizures in mice with rdTBI. Four of 9 (44%) mice developed recurrent spontaneous seizures; 3 (33%) mice developed convulsive seizures; 1 (11%) mouse developed recurrent spontaneous nonconvulsive seizures; and 5 of 9 (56%) mice had no seizures. (B) Electroencephalogram (EEG) trace of a 3xSham mouse 50 days after the electrode placement surgery. Channel (Ch) reading: right parietal electrode to left parietal electrode. (C) EEG trace of a mouse with a spontaneous convulsive seizure 35 days postinjury (dpi). The enlarged panel (with timescale 3 s) indicates emergence of high-amplitude evolving repetitive spikes and spike waves followed by postictal depression (right part of the enlarged panel). Channel reading as in b and (D) EEG traces of a nonconvulsive seizure at 65 dpi consisting of repetitive high-amplitude spike-and-slow-wave discharges in the absence of any movement of the mouse. Channel reading: Ch1 right frontal to left parietal electrode; Ch2 left parietal to right parietal electrode. (E) EEG power spectrum analysis of normal EEGs and convulsive and nonconvulsive seizures.

(Continued)

Following TBI, daily administration of levetiracetam, a commonly prescribed antiepileptic drug (AED), reduced IL-1β expression, cortical contusion volume, neuronal loss, and reversed TBI-induced GLT-1 loss 20 days following CCI in rats, suggesting that levetiracetam might have neuroprotective and antiepileptic effects postinjury [31] (Fig. 10.4). Mice treated with an IL-1 receptor antagonist showed reduced seizure susceptibility and reduction in hippocampal astrogliosis 2 weeks following injury compared with vehicle. Six months following injury, mice treated with the IL-1 receptor antagonist had fewer evoked seizures, decreased seizure severity, and a significantly lower seizure severity score [32] (Fig. 10.5). Administering antibodies against IL-1β significantly reduced TBI-induced loss of hippocampal neurons in a rat model of TBI [33]. In a comparable study, following FPI, mice had increased microglial activation, increased dopaminergic innervation, and decreased number of parvalbumin (PV)-positive interneurons in the globus pallidus [34]. Neutralization of IL-1β in these mice reduced microglial activation, normalized dopaminergic innervation, and prevented the loss of PV + interneurons [34]. Neutralization of IL-1β has also been shown to attenuate the loss of mature oligodendrocytes following diffuse TBI in mice [35]. Overall, these data suggest that targeting IL-1β following TBI could potentially be used to prevent the development of PTE.

Interleukin-10

IL-10 is an anti-inflammatory cytokine that can be produced by activated microglia and reactive astrocytes in the brain. Following TBI, IL-10 levels are elevated in the CSF of patients [36] whereas chronically reduced IL-10 plasma levels are lower in patients with temporal lobe epilepsy (TLE) + hippocampal sclerosis (HS) than in patients with TLE without HS [37]. Intravenous infusion and subcutaneous injection of IL-10 following TBI has been shown to improve neurological recovery and reduce levels of TNF-α in the rat FPI model [38]. In rat hippocampal slices, IL-10 application has also been shown to reduce epileptiform activity [39]. To our knowledge, no studies to date have shown whether IL-10 is regulated in PTE models. Based on TBI and epilepsy preclinical studies, IL-10 may be useful if therapeutically upregulated following TBI to reduce the risk of PTE.

FIG. 10.3, CONT'D The power density spectra are color-coded on a logarithmic scale (dB). Pink panels in c–e show the location of the ictal event in the EEG and in the corresponding power spectrum. (F) Seizure frequency in rdTBI mice with convulsive and nonconvulsive seizures compared with 3xSham. (G) Histological confirmation of the absence of gross tissue loss induced by either rdTBI or electrode placement surgery. (H) Diffuse loss of GLT-1 and Kir4.1 expression in astrocytes in mice with spontaneous recurrent seizures and I. quantification of GLT-1 loss. *$P \le .05$, **$P \le .01$. *(Reproduced with permission from Shandra O, et al. Repetitive diffuse mild traumatic brain injury causes an atypical astrocyte response and spontaneous recurrent seizures. J Neurosci 2019;39(10):1944–963.)*

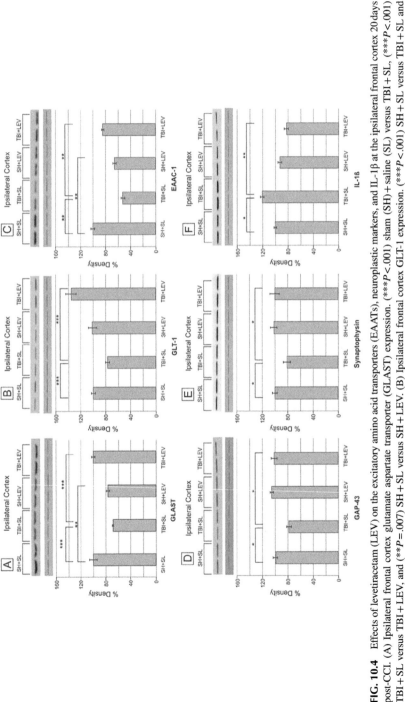

FIG. 10.4 Effects of levetiracetam (LEV) on the excitatory amino acid transporters (EAATs), neuroplastic markers, and IL-1β at the ipsilateral frontal cortex 20days post-CCI. (A) Ipsilateral frontal cortex glutamate aspartate transporter (GLAST) expression. (***P < .001) sham (SH) + saline (SL) versus TBI + SL, (***P < .001) TBI + SL versus TBI + LEV, and (**P = .007) SH + SL versus SH + LEV. (B) Ipsilateral frontal cortex GLT-1 expression. (***P < .001) SH + SL versus TBI + SL and (***P < .001) TBI + SL versus TBI + LEV. (C) Ipsilateral frontal cortex excitatory amino-acid carrier 1 (EAAC-1) expression. (***P < .001) SH + SL versus TBI + SL, (***P < .001) TBI + SL versus TBI + LEV, and (**P = .005). (D) Ipsilateral frontal cortex growth associated protein-43 (GAP-43) expression. (*P = .022) SH + SL versus TBI + SL and (**P = .017) TBI + SL versus TBI + LEV. (E) Ipsilateral frontal cortex synaptophysin expression. (*P = .024) SH + SL versus TBI + SL and (*P = .018) TBI + SL versus CCI + LEV. (F) Ipsilateral frontal cortex IL-1β expression. (*P = .035) SH + SL versus TBI + SL and (**P = .008) TBI + SL versus TBI + LEV. SH + SL indicates sham injured rats and daily saline administration; TBI + SL, traumatic brain injury rats and daily saline administration; SH + LEV, sham injured rats receiving daily levetiracetam; TBI + LEV, traumatic brain injury rats receiving daily levetiracetam administration. *(Reproduced with permission from Zou et al. Neuroprotective, neuroplastic, and neurobehavioral effects of daily treatment with levetiracetam in experimental traumatic brain injury. Neurorehabil Neural Repair 2013;27(9):878–88.)*

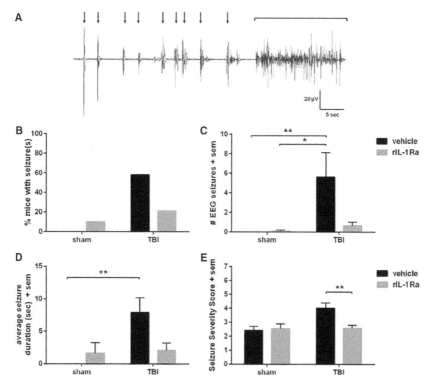

FIG. 10.5 Human acute recombinant IL-1 receptor antagonist (rIL-1Ra) treatment reduces the chronic evoked seizure response. (A) PTZ results in a stereotypical pattern of brief, abnormal epileptiform events paired with isolated myoclonic contractions *(black arrows)*, which was observed in some mice to culminate in a generalized convulsive seizure *(black bracket)*. (B) Fifty-eight percent of vehicle-TBI mice exhibited an evoked seizure in response to PTZ, compared with only 21% of IL-1Ra-TBI mice (Fisher's exact test, $P=.07$). (C) Quantification of EEG seizures (revealed an increase in vehicle-TBI mice but not in rIL-1Ra-TBI mice compared with their respective sham controls (Kruskal-Wallis test, $P<.01$; post hoc, $P<.01$), but no increase in rIL-1Ra-TBI mice compared with their sham controls. (D) Average seizure duration was similarly increased specifically in vehicle-TBI mice compared with sham controls ($P<.01$). (E) The overall seizure severity score revealed a significant effect of injury ($F(1,50)=4.96$, $P=.03$) and a treatment × injury interaction ($F(1,50)=4.65$, $P=.04$), with post hoc analysis finding an elevation only in vehicle-TBI mice compared with IL-1Ra-TBI mice ($P<.01$). $n=11$/group (sham) and 15–19/group (TBI); *$P<.05$, **$P<.01$. *(Reproduced with permission from Semple BD, et al. Interleukin-1 receptor in seizure susceptibility after traumatic injury to the pediatric brain. J Neurosci 2017;37(33):7864–877.)*

Tumor necrosis factor-alpha

TNF-α is a pleiotropic cytokine that can be produced by both activated microglia and astrocytes in the CNS following injury. TNF-α has been shown to be elevated in patients and preclinical models of TBI [40–42]. Treatment with etanercept, a TNF-α antagonist, has been shown to attenuate cerebral ischemia and increased levels of TNF-α following FPI in rats [43]. TNF-α expression is elevated up to 21 days after traumatic injury in organotypic hippocampal slice cultures [44]. Neutralizing TNF-α with a polyclonal antibody reduced ictal discharges whereas neutralizing interleukin-6 (IL-6) or treating with phenytoin was not successful in reducing the development of epileptiform activity [44]. Following CCI, TNF-α levels were also elevated at the site of injury 24 h postinjury [45]. Pretreatment with the Toll-like receptor (TLR) agonists, monophosphoryl lipid A (MPL), and tri-palmitoyl-S-glyceryl-cysteine (Pam3Cys) prevented the increase in TNF-α levels following trauma [45]. Rats pretreated with TLR agonists had significantly higher seizure thresholds when challenged with electrical stimuli compared to vehicle [45]. Inhibiting TLR-4 has also been shown to reduce brain edema and IL-6 production which is thought to be dependent on HMGB1 [46]. Taken together, these data suggest that suppression of TNF-α could be therapeutically targeted to reduce the development of PTE following brain injury.

Interleukin-6

IL-6 is a cytokine that has both pro-inflammatory and anti-inflammatory properties [47]. In the CNS, astrocytes and microglia are the primary sources of IL-6 while neurons can produce IL-6 during CNS disease and injury [48]. Elevated IL-6 levels have been documented following brain injury and were significantly elevated in patients that developed PTE [49,50]. When comparing adult patients with TBI, with seizures and without seizure, serum IL-6 levels were significantly higher in patients with PTE [49] (Fig. 10.6). This prospective study also analyzed the inflammatory markers TNF-α and interferon-gamma (IFN-γ) but did not observe a significant difference in serum levels between the seizure and nonseizure groups. These data demonstrate that IL-6 signaling could potentially be implicated in the development of PTE. Neutralization of IL-6, using an anti-IL-6 antibody, suppresses postinjury neuroinflammation and improves motor coordination in a mouse head injury model [50]. Transgenic mice that overexpress IL-6 develop spontaneous tonic-clonic seizures [51]. Conversely, studies have shown that IL-6 administration shortens hyperthermia-induced seizures in developing rats while exacerbating the severity of seizures in adult rats [52]. Interestingly, microglial IL-6 increases expression of astrocytic aquaporin-4 (AQP4) which could be implicated in edema following injury [46]. Systemic administration of an anti-IL-6 antibody has been shown to reverse neuronal injury and inflammation in the frontal cortex and hippocampus following mechanical ventilation-induced lung injury (VILI) in mice [53]. Future studies should determine whether IL-6 inhibition has neuroprotective and antiepileptogenic effects in PTE.

Transforming growth factor-beta

TGF-β is a cytokine produced by neural and glial cells in the CNS that play a role in cell proliferation, differentiation, and survival [54]. TGF-β signaling is increased after brain injury in patients and animal models of TBI [55,56].

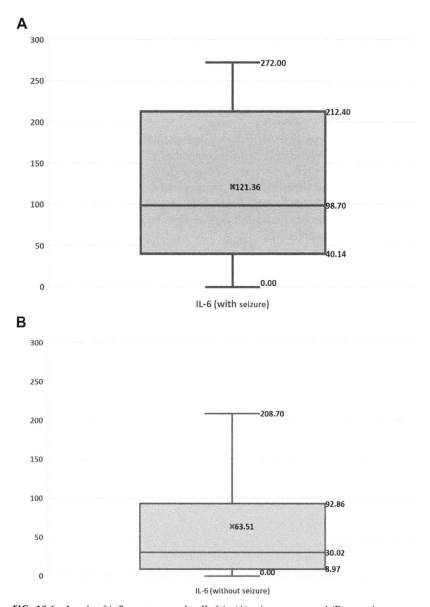

FIG. 10.6 Levels of inflammatory marker IL-6 in (A) seizure group and (B) nonseizure group. The center lines indicate medians, X indicates mean, boxes indicate 25th–75th percentiles, and whiskers indicate the minimum and maximum. Values are in pg/mL. *(Reproduced with permission from Choudhary A, et al. A prospective study of novel therapeutic targets interleukin-6, tumor necrosis factor alpha, and interferon gamma as predictive biomarkers for the development of posttraumatic epilepsy. World Neurosurg X 2021;12:100107.)*

TGF-β has been shown to cause the activation of IL-1β and TNF-α in rats after mild FPI. Further, inhibition of TGF-β reduces neuroinflammation and apoptosis after injury [55] (TGF-β/albumin involvement in PTE is discussed in Chapter 9). Further studies are needed to elucidate the role TGF-β may play in the development of PTE.

Migration inhibitory factor

The inflammatory cytokine MIF is elevated after TBI, and higher levels of MIF correlate with worse posttraumatic outcomes [57–59]. Elevated MIF has also been shown to affect neuronal function in the hippocampus. MIF applied acutely to mice brain slices increases frequency of calcium events in CA1 pyramidal neurons [57]. Inhibition of MIF following FPI reduces astrocyte activation but is not neuroprotective in the perilesional cortex [57]. Future studies should determine whether MIF antagonists display potential as therapies for prevention of PTE.

Neuroinflammation plays a critical role in the development of PTE following TBI. Following TBI, activated microglia and astrocytes can migrate to the site of injury and release both pro- and anti-inflammatory cytokines and chemokines. Chronic inflammation following TBI can be observed months to years after injury and could contribute to the development and/or maintenance of epilepsy. Clinical and preclinical evidence suggests that targeting neuroinflammation may be neuroprotective and antiepileptogenic. Inflammatory markers have been shown to be associated with increased risk of PTE over time, suggesting that cytokines could potentially be used as a biomarker to predict risk for development of PTE. Taken together, neuroinflammation plays a crucial role in brain homeostasis, and chronic inflammation may contribute to the development of PTE.

References

[1] Webster KM, et al. Inflammation in epileptogenesis after traumatic brain injury. J Neuroinflammation 2017;14(1):10.

[2] Ramlackhansingh AF, et al. Inflammation after trauma: microglial activation and traumatic brain injury. Ann Neurol 2011;70(3):374–83.

[3] van Vliet EA, et al. Long-lasting blood-brain barrier dysfunction and neuroinflammation after traumatic brain injury. Neurobiol Dis 2020;145, 105080.

[4] Vezzani A, et al. The role of inflammation in epilepsy. Nat Rev Neurol 2011;7(1):31–40.

[5] Saletti PG, et al. In search of antiepileptogenic treatments for post-traumatic epilepsy. Neurobiol Dis 2019;123:86–99.

[6] DiSabato DJ, Quan N, Godbout JP. Neuroinflammation: the devil is in the details. J Neurochem 2016;139(Suppl 2):136–53.

[7] Kumar A, et al. Microglial/macrophage polarization dynamics following traumatic brain injury. J Neurotrauma 2016;33(19):1732–50.

[8] Olah M, et al. Microglia phenotype diversity. CNS Neurol Disord Drug Targets 2011;10(1):108–18.

[9] Loane DJ, Kumar A. Microglia in the TBI brain: the good, the bad, and the dysregulated. Exp Neurol 2016;275(Pt 3):316–27.

[10] Kan M, et al. Circulating high mobility group box-1 and toll-like receptor 4 expressions increase the risk and severity of epilepsy. Braz J Med Biol Res 2019;52(7), e7374.

[11] Han Y, et al. HMGB1/CXCL12-mediated immunity and Th17 cells might underlie highly suspected autoimmune epilepsy in elderly individuals. Neuropsychiatr Dis Treat 2020;16:1285–93.

[12] Webster KM, et al. Targeting high-mobility group box protein 1 (HMGB1) in pediatric traumatic brain injury: chronic neuroinflammatory, behavioral, and epileptogenic consequences. Exp Neurol 2019;320, 112979.

[13] Di Sapia R, et al. In-depth characterization of a mouse model of post-traumatic epilepsy for biomarker and drug discovery. Acta Neuropathol Commun 2021;9(1):76.

[14] Gordon S. Alternative activation of macrophages. Nat Rev Immunol 2003;3(1):23–35.

[15] Okuneva O, et al. Abnormal microglial activation in the Cstb(−/−) mouse, a model for progressive myoclonus epilepsy, EPM1. Glia 2015;63(3):400–11.

[16] Therajaran P, et al. Microglial polarization in posttraumatic epilepsy: potential mechanism and treatment opportunity. Epilepsia 2020;61(2):203–15.

[17] Robinson C, Apgar C, Shapiro LA. Astrocyte hypertrophy contributes to aberrant neurogenesis after traumatic brain injury. Neural Plast 2016;2016:1347987.

[18] Danzer SC. Contributions of adult-generated granule cells to hippocampal pathology in temporal lobe epilepsy: a neuronal bestiary. Brain Plast 2018;3(2):169–81.

[19] Ribak CE, et al. Seizure-induced formation of basal dendrites on granule cells of the rodent dentate gyrus. In: Noebels JL, et al., editors. Jasper's Basic Mechanisms of the Epilepsies. Bethesda, MD: National Center for Biotechnology Information; 2012.

[20] Shandra O, et al. Repetitive diffuse mild traumatic brain injury causes an atypical astrocyte response and spontaneous recurrent seizures. J Neurosci 2019;39(10):1944–63.

[21] Arulsamy A, Shaikh MF. Tumor necrosis factor-alpha, the pathological key to post-traumatic epilepsy: a comprehensive systematic review. ACS Chem Nerosci 2020;11(13):1900–8.

[22] Youn Y, Sung IK, Lee IG. The role of cytokines in seizures: interleukin (IL)-1beta, IL-1Ra, IL-8, and IL-10. Korean J Pediatr 2013;56(7):271–4.

[23] Paudel YN, et al. HMGB1: a common biomarker and potential target for TBI, neuroinflammation, epilepsy, and cognitive dysfunction. Front Neurosci 2018;12:628.

[24] Balosso S, et al. Tumor necrosis factor-alpha inhibits seizures in mice via p75 receptors. Ann Neurol 2005;57(6):804–12.

[25] Balosso S, et al. The dual role of TNF-alpha and its receptors in seizures. Exp Neurol 2013;247:267–71.

[26] Patel DC, et al. Hippocampal TNF-alpha signaling contributes to seizure generation in an infection-induced mouse model of limbic epilepsy. eNeuro 2017;4(2).

[27] Zhu G, et al. Effects of interleukin-1beta on hippocampal glutamate and GABA releases associated with Ca2+−induced Ca2+ releasing systems. Epilepsy Res 2006;71(2–3):107–16.

[28] Diamond ML, et al. IL-1beta associations with posttraumatic epilepsy development: a genetics and biomarker cohort study. Epilepsia 2014;55(7):1109–19.

[29] Darrah SD, et al. Genetic variability in glutamic acid decarboxylase genes: associations with post-traumatic seizures after severe TBI. Epilepsy Res 2013;103(2–3):180–94.

[30] Wagner AK, et al. Adenosine A1 receptor gene variants associated with post-traumatic seizures after severe TBI. Epilepsy Res 2010;90(3):259–72.

[31] Zou H, et al. Neuroprotective, neuroplastic, and neurobehavioral effects of daily treatment with levetiracetam in experimental traumatic brain injury. Neurorehabil Neural Repair 2013;27(9):878–88.

[32] Semple BD, et al. Interleukin-1 receptor in seizure susceptibility after traumatic injury to the pediatric brain. J Neurosci 2017;37(33):7864–77.

[33] Lu KT, et al. Effect of interleukin-1 on traumatic brain injury-induced damage to hippocampal neurons. J Neurotrauma 2005;22(8):885–95.

[34] Ozen I, et al. Interleukin-1 beta neutralization attenuates traumatic brain injury-induced microglia activation and neuronal changes in the globus pallidus. Int J Mol Sci 2020;21(2).

[35] Flygt J, et al. Neutralization of interleukin-1beta following diffuse traumatic brain injury in the mouse attenuates the loss of mature oligodendrocytes. J Neurotrauma 2018;35(23):2837–49.

[36] Bell MJ, et al. Interleukin-6 and interleukin-10 in cerebrospinal fluid after severe traumatic brain injury in children. J Neurotrauma 1997;14(7):451–7.

[37] Basnyat P, et al. Chronically reduced IL-10 plasma levels are associated with hippocampal sclerosis in temporal lobe epilepsy patients. BMC Neurol 2020;20(1):241.

[38] Knoblach SM, Faden AI. Interleukin-10 improves outcome and alters proinflammatory cytokine expression after experimental traumatic brain injury. Exp Neurol 1998;153(1):143–51.

[39] Levin SG, Godukhin OV. Protective effects of interleukin-10 on the development of epileptiform activity evoked by transient episodes of hypoxia in rat hippocampal slices. Neurosci Behav Physiol 2007;37(5):467–70.

[40] Goodman JC, et al. Elevation of tumor necrosis factor in head injury. J Neuroimmunol 1990;30(2–3):213–7.

[41] Ross SA, et al. The presence of tumour necrosis factor in CSF and plasma after severe head injury. Br J Neurosurg 1994;8(4):419–25.

[42] Taupin V, et al. Increase in IL-6, IL-1 and TNF levels in rat brain following traumatic lesion. Influence of pre- and post-traumatic treatment with Ro5 4864, a peripheral-type (p site) benzodiazepine ligand. J Neuroimmunol 1993;42(2):177–85.

[43] Chio CC, et al. Etanercept attenuates traumatic brain injury in rats by reducing early microglial expression of tumor necrosis factor-alpha. BMC Neurosci 2013;14:33.

[44] Chong SA, et al. Intrinsic inflammation is a potential anti-epileptogenic target in the organotypic hippocampal slice model. Neurotherapeutics 2018;15(2):470–88.

[45] Hesam S, et al. Monophosphoryl lipid A and Pam3Cys prevent the increase in seizure susceptibility and epileptogenesis in rats undergoing traumatic brain injury. Neurochem Res 2018;43(10):1978–85.

[46] Laird MD, et al. High mobility group box protein-1 promotes cerebral edema after traumatic brain injury via activation of toll-like receptor 4. Glia 2014;62(1):26–38.

[47] Wolf J, Rose-John S, Garbers C. Interleukin-6 and its receptors: a highly regulated and dynamic system. Cytokine 2014;70(1):11–20.

[48] Gruol DL. IL-6 regulation of synaptic function in the CNS. Neuropharmacology 2015;96(Pt A):42–54.

[49] Choudhary A, et al. A prospective study of novel therapeutic targets interleukin 6, tumor necrosis factor alpha, and interferon gamma as predictive biomarkers for the development of posttraumatic epilepsy. World Neurosurg X 2021;12, 100107.

[50] Yang SH, et al. Interleukin 6 mediates neuroinflammation and motor coordination deficits after mild traumatic brain injury and brief hypoxia in mice. Shock 2013;40(6):471–5.

[51] Campbell IL, et al. Neurologic disease induced in transgenic mice by cerebral overexpression of interleukin 6. Proc Natl Acad Sci U S A 1993;90(21):10061–5.

[52] Fukuda M, et al. Interleukin-6 attenuates hyperthermia-induced seizures in developing rats. Brain Dev 2007;29(10):644–8.

[53] Sparrow NA, et al. IL-6 inhibition reduces neuronal injury in a murine model of ventilator-induced lung injury. Am J Respir Cell Mol Biol 2021;65(4):403–12.

[54] Pratt BM, McPherson JM. TGF-beta in the central nervous system: potential roles in ischemic injury and neurodegenerative diseases. Cytokine Growth Factor Rev 1997;8(4):267–92.

[55] Patel RK, et al. Transforming growth factor-beta 1 signaling regulates neuroinflammation and apoptosis in mild traumatic brain injury. Brain Behav Immun 2017;64:244–58.

[56] Morganti-Kossmann MC, et al. TGF-beta is elevated in the CSF of patients with severe traumatic brain injuries and parallels blood-brain barrier function. J Neurotrauma 1999;16(7):617–28.

[57] Newell-Rogers MK, et al. Antagonism of macrophage migration inhibitory factory (MIF) after traumatic brain injury ameliorates astrocytosis and peripheral lymphocyte activation and expansion. Int J Mol Sci 2020;21(20).

[58] Dai JX, et al. Utility of serum macrophage migration inhibitory factor as a potential biomarker for detection of cerebrocardiac syndrome following severe traumatic brain injury. Clin Chim Acta 2021;512:179–84.

[59] Yang DB, et al. Serum macrophage migration inhibitory factor concentrations correlate with prognosis of traumatic brain injury. Clin Chim Acta 2017;469:99–104.

Chapter 11

Biomarkers and treatment trials in animal models to prevent posttraumatic epilepsy

Overview

Investigating biomarkers and potential therapies in animal models is essential to determine which target mechanisms could prevent posttraumatic epilepsy (PTE). In theory, an ideal candidate biomarker should be easily measurable (noninvasive) and specific for PTE (distinct from traumatic brain injury (TBI) and epilepsy biomarkers) while an ideal therapeutic agent would be efficacious at preventing the development of seizures and secondary injuries associated with brain injury. In this chapter, we will discuss biomarkers and therapeutic interventions that reduce seizure susceptibility examined in animal models of PTE.

Biomarkers

Biomarkers reviewed here have been observed in animal models of TBI with documented incidence of PTE.

Imaging biomarkers

Magnetic resonance imaging (MRI) is a noninvasive tool that is utilized for many diagnoses, including locating epileptic foci and identifying abnormalities in patients following TBI [1,2]. In an MRI study using lateral fluid percussion injury (LFPI) in rats, Shultz *et al.* conducted T2-weighted image (T2WI) scans to examine large-deformation, high-dimensional mapping of hippocampal morphometry (HDM-LD). HDM-LD analysis revealed that lateral regions of the hippocampus were increased (thicker) in the animals that developed PTE, whereas the medial-ventral regions were decreased (thinner) in the animals that did not develop PTE [3] (Fig. 11.1). In a controlled cortical impact (CCI) injury study, T2WI analysis revealed a reduction in cortical volume at 3 months postinjury in mice that developed PTE compared to controls. No volumetric changes were observed in the hippocampus and striatum of PTE and no-SRS (spontaneous recurrent seizure) mice compared to controls. Quantification of

Posttraumatic Epilepsy. https://doi.org/10.1016/B978-0-323-90099-7.00010-1

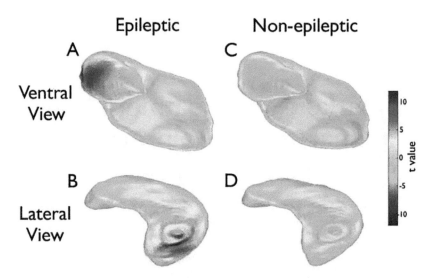

FIG. 11.1 Large-deformation, high-dimensional mapping (HDM-LD) of the ipsilateral hippocampus illustrating changes in epileptic (A and B) and nonepileptic rats (C and D) 1 week after lateral fluid percussion injury (LFPI) compared to baseline. Epileptic rats displayed significantly thicker surface in the lateral region of the hippocampus at one-week post-LFPI *(red-yellow)* compared to baseline. Statistical significance between the groups: $P < .05$ (unpaired two-tailed t-test, corrected for multiple comparisons). Nonepileptic rats displayed significantly thinner surface in the medial-ventral region at 1 week post-LFPI *(blue)* compared to baseline. *(Reproduced with permission from Shultz SR, et al. Can structural or functional changes following traumatic brain injury in the rat predict epileptic outcome? Epilepsia 2013;54(7):1240–250.)*

neuronal cell loss in the hemisphere contralateral to the impact showed cortical and hippocampal neurodegeneration in PTE mice, but not in no-SRS mice [4]. These findings suggest that MRI scans may potentially detect subtle changes or mechanisms involved in the development of PTE. In a different imaging study, using T_2 relaxation and diffusion tensor MRI at early time points following TBI, the severity of acute thalamic damage could differentiate animals that develop epilepsy from those that do not in the rat LFPI model [5]. These data suggest that thalamic damage could potentially be used as a prognostic biomarker for PTE. Taken together, MRI has also been utilized in animal models to identify imaging biomarkers for PTE that could aid in early diagnosis.

Protein biomarkers

Interleukin-1 beta (IL-1β) levels are elevated following brain injury, suggesting that it might be a useful biomarker for PTE [6,7]. Higher cerebrospinal fluid (CSF)/serum IL-1β ratios collected during the first week postinjury are associated with increased risk for PTE [7]. Mice treated with an IL-1 receptor antagonist also have reduced seizure susceptibility when challenged with pentylenetetrazol (PTZ) [8] (Chapter 10), suggesting that IL-1β could be a potential biomarker and therapeutic target for PTE; however, future studies are needed to determine whether IL-1β inhibition can prevent the development of unprovoked spontaneous seizures following brain injury.

Matrix metalloproteinases (MMPs) have been shown to modulate blood-brain barrier integrity through digestion and remodeling of extracellular matrix (ECM) proteins (Chapter 9). Elevation of MMP-9 levels has been shown to promote epileptogenesis after brain injury in the CCI model [9]. Serum MMP-9 levels are elevated acutely in patients following TBI [10]. To our knowledge, retrospective studies have not been performed to determine whether there is a difference in serum MMP levels in patients who develop PTE compared to those who do not, but clearly MMPs warrant further investigation.

Postinjury weight loss

One study suggests that weight loss could potentially be used as a biomarker to predict PTE development [11]. Following LFPI in rats, the mean weight of animals is reduced during the first week postinjury and then increases. Interestingly, mean body weight is significantly lower in TBI rats that develop epilepsy than in TBI rats that do not develop epilepsy. Specifically, body weight in the TBI group with epilepsy was significantly lower on days 4, 6, 7, 14, and 35 postinjury [11]. In addition, the group did not observe a difference in behavioral and cognitive outcomes in TBI rats that developed epilepsy compared with TBI rats that did not at various time points postinjury. These data suggest that differences in body weight following TBI could be used as a predictive marker for PTE but should be used with caution since weight loss can also occur secondary to numerous diseases (gastrointestinal diseases, endocrine disorders) [12,13].

Electrophysiological biomarkers

High-frequency oscillations (HFOs) are fast local oscillatory field potentials of frequency > 80 Hz, commonly subdivided into ripples (80–250 Hz) and fast ripples (>250 Hz). HFOs have served as a biomarker in human epilepsy [14] and have also been reported in animal models of TBI [15]. In the LFPI model, Li et al. observed higher (faster) mean peak frequency of ripple (80–200 Hz) rates in mice that developed PTE compared to mice that did not develop PTE. This increase was found in regions both ipsilateral and contralateral to the lesion with rate differences most significant in the perilesional site, the homotopic contralateral site, and bilateral hippocampi. Increased fast ripple (FR, 250–500 Hz) rates were also reported in PTE mice and remained stable throughout the duration of the experiment compared to nonepileptic mice [16] (Table 11.1). These results indicate that ripple rates may serve as a temporary biomarker for PTE, while fast ripple rates may serve as a more stable biomarker.

TABLE 11.1 Descriptive statistics of HFO occurrence rates (num/min) in control (sham), $E-$ (nonepileptic), and $E+$ (epileptic) groups.

Event type		Sham (n = 8)	$E-$ (n = 18)	$E+$ (n = 22)
HFO	Total numbers	16,858	53,622	133,070
	Mean (SD)	1.00 (1.32)	1.81 (2.21)	3.64 (3.48)
	Range (min, max)	(0, 9.07)	(0, 14.46)	(0, 14.68)
Ripple	Total numbers	14,895	44,755	91,224
	Mean (SD)	0.88 (1.23)	1.53 (2.04)	2.52 (2.67)
	Range (min, max)	(0, 9.05)	(0, 14.03)	(0, 14.22)
Fast ripple	Total numbers	1963	8867	41,846
	Mean (SD)	0.11 (0.19)	0.28 (0.38)	1.11 (1.2784)
	Range (min, max)	(0, 1.42)	(0, 2.34)	(0, 6.9513)

Reproduced with permission from Li L, Kumar U, You J, Zhou Y, Weiss SA, Bragin A. Spatial and temporal profile of high-frequency oscillations in posttraumatic epileptogenesis. Neurobiol Dis 2021;161:105544.

Treatment trials

Treatment trials in animal models of TBI are critical in order to determine potential therapeutic targets for both the prevention and the treatment of PTE (Table 11.2).

Baicalein

Ferroptosis is a lipid-peroxidation-dependent form of nonapoptotic oxidative cell death that could be involved in the development of PTE [17,26,27]. Pretreatment with baicalein, a flavonoid compound shown to inhibit ferroptosis, reduces seizure score, number of seizures, and average seizure duration in the iron chloride ($FeCl_3$)-induced model of PTE [17]. Pretreatment with baicalein also attenuates neuronal damage in an *in vitro* iron-induced neuronal injury model using $FeCl_3$ [17]. HT22 hippocampal neurons pretreated with baicalein have increased cell viability, measured with CCK8 assay, compared to nontreated cells [17]. Pretreatment daily with Lipo-1, a specific inhibitor of ferroptosis, also reduced seizure score in the $FeCl_3$-induced model of PTE [17]. These data suggest that inhibition of ferroptosis could exert neuroprotective and antiseizure effects in the $FeCl_3$-induced model of PTE. One caveat to this study is that pretreatment with a therapeutic agent does not translate into treatment in a clinical setting following injury. Future studies should determine whether treatment with ferroptosis inhibitors following brain injury has neuroprotective and/or antiepileptic effects in mechanical models of TBI.

TABLE 11.2 Treatment trials in animal models of PTE.

Treatment	Model/species	Dosage	Target/mechanism of action	Outcome	Reference
Baicalein	Iron chloride (FeCl$_3$)-induced PTE/mouse	50 and 100 mg/kg 30 min prior to FeCl$_3$ administration	Inhibits lipoxygenases (inhibiting 12/15-LOX-mediated lipid peroxidation), inhibits ferroptosis	Reduces seizure score, number of seizures, and average seizure duration	[17]
Lipo-1	Iron chloride (FeCl$_3$)-induced PTE/mouse	10 mg/kg/day 3 days prior to FeCl$_3$ administration	Ferroptosis inhibitor	Reduces seizure score	[17]
Brivaracetam	FPI/rat	650 mg/kg/day 30 min, 4 h or 8 h post-TBI for 5 days followed by oral administration in drinking water available ad libitum for 4 weeks	Targets SV2A which prevents synaptic vesicle exocytosis and release of excitatory neurotransmitters	Reduces overall seizure incidence, seizure frequency, time spent seizing, and spreading seizures	[18]
Ceftriaxone	FPI/rat	200 mg/kg/day for 7 days post-TBI	Transcriptional enhancer of glutamate transporter-1	Reduces seizure frequency, total ictal time	[19]
Rapamycin	CCI/mouse	6 mg/kg/day 1 h post-TBI and once daily up to 4 weeks	mTOR inhibitor	Reduces overall seizure incidence, seizure frequency	[20]
Sodium selenate	FPI/rat	1 mg/kg/day for 4 weeks	Activation of protein phosphatase 2A (PP2A), reduces levels of hyperphosphorylated tau	Reduces number of seizures per day, seizure duration	[21]
SR141716A	FPI/rat	z or 10 mg/kg (data were combined for both doses) within 2 min post-TBI	CB1 receptor antagonist	Prevents long-term increase in seizure susceptibility following brain injury	[22]
Atipamezole	FPI/rat	100 μg/kg/h 7 days post-TBI and continued for 9 weeks	α$_2$-adrenoceptor antagonist	Reduces seizure susceptibility	[23]
Minozac	CCI/mouse	5 mg/kg 3 h and 6 h post-TBI	Selective inhibitor of pro-inflammatory cytokines released by activated glia	Reduces seizure susceptibility	[24]
TAK242	Undercut/mouse	3 mg/kg/day 1 day post-TBI for 1 week	TLR4 antagonist	Reduces seizure susceptibility	[25]
RAGE monoclonal antibody	Undercut/mouse	10 mg/kg/day 1 day post-TBI for 1 week	Inhibits RAGE	Reduces seizure susceptibility	[25]

FPI, fluid percussion injury; CCI, controlled cortical impact.

Brivaracetam

Brivaracetam, a derivative of levetiracetam, binds to synaptic vesicle protein 2A (SV2A) in the brain which prevents synaptic vesicle exocytosis and release of excitatory neurotransmitters in the synaptic cleft [28]. Brivaracetam treatment following brain injury reduces the overall incidence of seizures and seizure frequency compared to saline-injected controls in the rostral parasagittal fluid percussion injury (rpFPI) rat model [18]. *Ex vivo* neocortical slices of rats treated with brivaracetam 3–4 weeks postinjury also show reduced evoked and spontaneous epileptiform activity compared to vehicle-treated animals [29]. Taken together, these data suggest that targeting SV2A following brain injury could potentially be used to prevent or reduce the occurrence of PTE, but comprehensive studies, including long-term continuous electroencephalogram (EEG) evaluation, need to be performed.

Ceftriaxone

Ceftriaxone is a β-lactam antibiotic that has neuroprotective effects in many animal models of neurological disease [30,31]. Ceftriaxone has been shown to increase levels of the glutamate transporter glutamate transporter-1 (GLT-1) in rodents and in human cultured astrocytes [19,32]. Glutamate transporter dysregulation can be observed following TBI in parallel to a decrease in glutamate clearance which could contribute to the development of epilepsy [33]. Treating rats with ceftriaxone daily postinjury restores GLT-1 expression in the lesioned cortex compared to vehicle-treated animals following fluid percussion injury (FPI) [19]. Ceftriaxone treatment following brain injury also reduces early posttraumatic seizures [19]. Rats treated with ceftriaxone have a reduction in seizure frequency and total ictal time compared to vehicle-treated animals 12 weeks postinjury [19]. These data suggest that early intervention with ceftriaxone postinjury could be used as a treatment to prevent or reduce PTE. It is important to note that there has been conflicting evidence in the field on whether ceftriaxone is a transcriptional activator of GLT-1 or whether modulation of GLT-1 is an off-target effect of treatment [34,35].

Rapamycin

Mammalian target of rapamycin (mTOR) signaling regulates multiple functions in the brain including neurogenesis, synaptic plasticity, and ion channel expression [36]. Hyperactivation of mTOR signaling can be observed following brain injury and in epilepsy which could be implemented in epileptogenesis [20,37]. The mTOR inhibitor rapamycin could have therapeutic effects in the prevention of PTE [20]. Rapamycin treatment in mice following CCI injury significantly decreased the development of PTE (Fig. 11.2) [20]. Additionally, rapamycin-treated mice that developed PTE had significantly fewer seizures per day than mice treated with vehicle [20]. Daily treatment with rapamycin following injury also reduced mossy fiber sprouting and neuronal degeneration in the hippocampus 3 days postinjury [20]. Taken together, these data suggest that

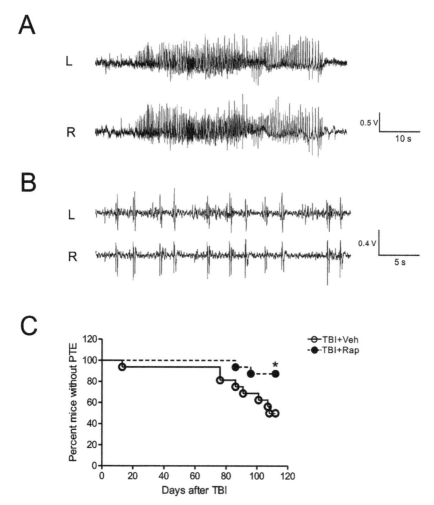

FIG. 11.2 Rapamycin attenuates development of posttraumatic epilepsy in the CCI model. (A) Representative EEG tracings of seizures. (B) Representative EEG tracings of interictal epileptiform abnormalities. (C) Rapamycin treatment significantly decreased the development of PTE following TBI. Statistical significances between the groups: * $P < .05$ (Mantel-Cox log-rank test). *(Reproduced with permission from Guo D, et al. Rapamycin attenuates the development of posttraumatic epilepsy in a mouse model of traumatic brain injury. PLoS One 2013;8(5):e64078.)*

inhibition of mTOR hyperactivation could have neuroprotective and antiepileptogenic effects following brain injury.

Sodium selenate

Tau proteins are important for the stabilization of microtubules in neurons in the central nervous system (CNS) [38]. Hyperphosphorylation of tau can be observed in patients and animal models of epilepsy which could induce neuronal dysfunction and death [39–41]. Expression of hyperphosphorylated-tau (p-tau) is increased in rats following FPI and has been observed in human TBI brain tissue [42]. Sodium selenate has been shown to reduce levels of p-tau through activation of protein phosphatase 2A (PP2A), a protein essential for the dephosphorylation of tau [43]. Rats treated with sodium selenate following FPI had a significantly lower number of seizures per day and shorter average seizure duration than vehicle-treated rats 12–14 weeks postinjury [21]. In contrast, sodium selenate did not reduce early seizure activity immediately following FPI, suggesting that sodium selenate may selectively reduce late seizures that occur as a result of PTE. These data suggest that hyperphosphorylation of tau might play an important role in PTE and could be targeted to reduce the severity of epilepsy following brain injury.

"Two-hit" injury models

In two-hit injury models, seizure susceptibility is assessed by challenging animals with a stimulus to induce seizures following brain injury [22–24]. Measurable outcomes include seizure latency, total seizure time, % of animals with seizures, and epileptiform discharges (EDs) [22–24]. The ideal model would examine which target mechanisms prevent the development of spontaneous seizures following traumatic injury, without proconvulsant intervention to induce seizures.

Cannabinoid type-1 receptor antagonist

Cannabinoid type-1 (CB1) receptor signaling could play a role in the development of epilepsy [44,45]. CB1 receptor blockade has been shown to have antiseizure effects in animal models of epilepsy [46]. The CB1 receptor antagonist SR141716A (rimonabant) could prevent seizure susceptibility following brain injury [22]. Rats that received a single dose of SR within 2 min of injury have increased seizure latency and decreased total seizure time compared to vehicle when challenged with kainic acid 6 weeks after FPI [22] (Fig. 11.3). Seizure susceptibility in SR-treated rats was comparable to noninjured sham controls, which suggests that CB1 receptor inhibition following brain injury might prevent long-term posttraumatic hyperexcitability [22]. Interestingly, administering SR 20 min following injury did not exert antiseizure effects compared to vehicle, measured by seizure latency and total seizure time when challenged with kainic acid, which suggests a narrow therapeutic time window [22]. However, in a different study, SR141716A treatment did not have antiepileptogenic effects following LFP in rats [23]. SR141716A administration 2 min post-TBI as a single dose or initiated 30 min postinjury continuously for 9 weeks did not prevent the development of epilepsy and did not decrease seizure susceptibility in mice challenged with PTZ 14 weeks postinjury [23]. Taken together, these conflicting results leave the role of CB1 receptors following TBI unclear.

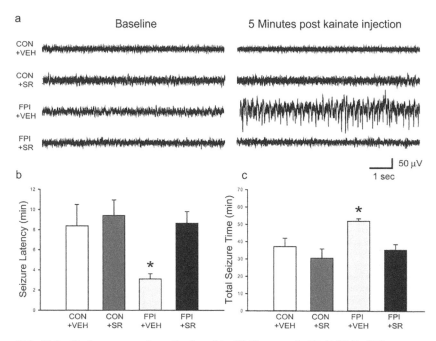

FIG. 11.3 Single posttraumatic application of the CB1R antagonist SR 141716A (SR) prevents the long-term increase in seizure susceptibility after brain trauma. Seizure susceptibility testing with kainate 6 weeks after fluid percussion injury (FPI) reveals increased seizure susceptibility in the head-injured, vehicle-treated (FPI + VEH) animals ($n = 14$) compared to the sham-injured, vehicle-treated (CON + VEH) animals ($n = 6$; $P = .022$ seizure latency, $P = .024$ seizure duration), but not in the head-injured, SR-treated (FPI + SR) animals ($n = 17$; $P = 1.00$ seizure latency, $P = .996$ seizure duration; SR injection within 2 min after FPI). Note that SR injection (2 min after sham injury) had no effect on the control animals (CON + SR; $n = 8$; $P = .986$ seizure latency, $P = .655$ seizure duration). (A) Representative traces from hippocampal depth EEG recordings made during baseline recording or 5 min after injection of kainate. (B) FPI results in a significant decrease in seizure latency, and this decrease is eliminated by posttraumatic injection of SR. (C) FPI results in a significant increase in the cumulative duration of the seizures, and this increase is eliminated by posttraumatic injection of SR. Statistical significant difference from CON + VEH: * $P < .05$ (one-way ANOVA followed by a Dunnett's *post hoc* test). Error bars: SEM. *(Reproduced with permission from Echegoyen J, et al. Single application of a CB1 receptor antagonist rapidly following head injury prevents long-term hyperexcitability in a rat model. Epilepsy Res 2009;85(1):123–27.)*

Atipamezole

Atipamezole (ATI) is a selective α_2-adrenoreceptor antagonist that has been shown to have both antiepileptic and proepileptic effects [47,48]. Rats treated with ATI starting at 7 days post-FPI and continued for 9 weeks have reduced seizure susceptibility and improved recovery after TBI compared to vehicle-treated controls [23]. Time to the 1st spike and the number of EDs after the administration of PTZ was normalized in rats treated with ATI initiated at 7 days postinjury [23] (Fig. 11.4). Interestingly, ATI treatment initiated 30 min following injury

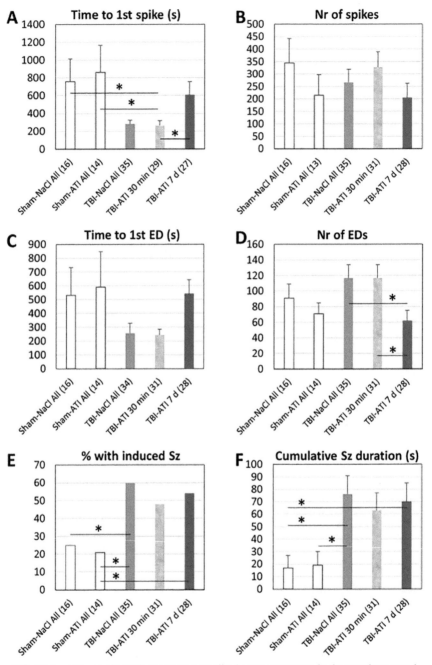

FIG. 11.4 Atipamezole (ATI) treatment normalized some parameters in the pentylenetetrazol (PTZ) seizure susceptibility test when assessed at 14 week (ATI 30 min treatment arm) or 15 week (ATI 7 day treatment arm) post-TBI. As the data in the Sham-NaCl 30 min and 7 day groups or in the Sham-ATI 30 min and 7 day groups did not differ, they were combined, and the new groups were named Sham-NaCl All and Sham-ATI All, respectively. (A) Time to the 1st spike after PTZ administration was normalized in the ATI 7 day treatment arm, indicating an antiepileptogenic effect of ATI (Kruskal-Wallis $P < .05$). (B) The number of spikes was reduced in the TBI-ATI 7 day group compared with that in the TBI-ATI 30 min group (Mann-Whitney U test $P < .05$).

(Continued)

did not reduce seizure susceptibility in rats when challenged with PTZ [23]. ATI did not prevent the development of epilepsy and did not reduce cumulative seizure duration in rats during the PTZ seizure susceptibility test. ATI treatment following FPI improved motor performance in rats, measured by the beam-walking test, but had no effect on spatial memory performance, measured by the Morris water maze, compared to vehicle [23]. Therefore, ATI might improve motor outcome when chronically administered after injury but does not prevent the development of epilepsy.

Minozac

Administration of the small-molecule minozac (Mzc) has been shown to suppress the upregulation of pro-inflammatory cytokines produced by activated glia and improve long-term neurologic outcome in mice following TBI [49]. One week following CCI injury, mice have increased seizure susceptibility in response to graded electroconvulsive shock (ECS) compared to sham [24] (Fig. 11.5). Treatment with Mzc, given as 2 doses 3 and 6 h postinjury, prevents this increase in seizure susceptibility, measured as seizure scores [24]. These data suggest that suppressing pro-inflammatory cytokine production might have some antiseizure effects, but this needs to be further evaluated in a chronic model of PTE.

High-mobility group box protein 1

High-mobility group box protein 1 (HMGB1) is a DNA-binding protein that plays a key role in neuroinflammation following TBI and epilepsy (Chapter 10). Activation of Toll-like receptor 4 (TLR4) and receptor for advanced glycation end products (RAGE) by HMGB1 could be involved in epileptogenesis [50–52]. In the undercut mouse model of TBI, expression of TLR4 and RAGE is increased in neurons, microglia, and endothelial cells in the cortex [25]. Undercut mice treated with TAK242, a TLR4 inhibitor, or a RAGE monoclonal antibody (mAb) have higher seizure thresholds than saline-treated undercut mice when challenged with PTZ [25]. Treatment with TAK242 or RAGE mAb reduced gliosis and ameliorated the loss of cortical neurons observed in saline-treated undercut mice. Additionally, undercut mice treated with TAK242 also had a

FIG. 11.4, CONT'D (C) The time to the 1st ED was normalized in the ATI 7-day treatment arm compared with the TBI-NaCl All or TBI-ATI 30 min groups (Mann-Whitney U test, both $P<.05$). (D) The number of epileptiform discharges (EDs) was normalized in the ATI 7 day treatment arm (Kruskal-Wallis $P<.05$). (E) Percentage of animals showing behavioral seizures (Sz) in the PTZ-test. As expected, a higher percentage of TBI animals exhibited induced seizures compared with the sham-injured groups, which was not affected by ATI. (F) Cumulative seizure duration in the PTZ-test was increased in TBI rats and was not alleviated by ATI (Kruskal-Wallis $P<.05$). The X-axis shows the animal groups. Number of animals is shown in parentheses. Data are shown as mean ± standard error of the mean (panels A, B, C, D, F). Statistical significances between the groups: * $P<.05$ (Mann-Whitney U test). *(Reproduced with permission from Nissinen J, et al. Disease-modifying effect of atipamezole in a model of posttraumatic epilepsy. Epilepsy Res 2017;136:18–34.)*

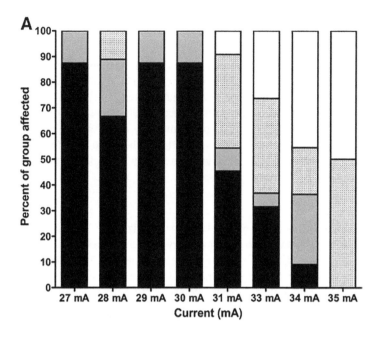

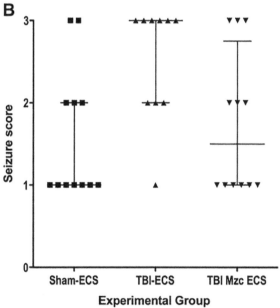

FIG. 11.5 Minozac treatment reduces seizure score in a "two-hit" injury model. (A) Stacked bar graph of responses to graded electroconvulsive shock (ECS) in naïve male CD1 mice. Mice were exposed to a single ECS in 1-mA increments from 27 to 35 mA ($n=8$–19 per group). The response to ECS was videotaped and scored by separate observers as either no response *(black)*, forelimb clonic seizure *(gray)*, fore and hind limb generalized tonic-clonic seizure (stippled), or death *(white)*. The seizure threshold was determined to be 30 mA ($\chi^2 P < .0001$ for 30 versus 31 mA). (B) Scatterplot of seizure scores (1, no seizure; 2, decreased activity; 3, forelimb or hind limb clonic seizure) following 30-mA ECS-induced seizure on day 7 after TBI (TBI-ECS),

(Continued)

significantly lower frequency of SRS compared to saline-treated undercut mice [25]. These data suggest that the TLR4 and RAGE pathways are involved in post-traumatic epileptogenesis and could potentially be targeted for PTE treatment.

Biomarkers and treatment trials in animal models are critical to identify potential therapeutic targets to prevent the development of epilepsy following brain injury. Multiple studies show that early intervention with therapeutic agents can reduce the occurrence of spontaneous seizures following injury. Biomarkers that identify early risk for the development of PTE may allow for prophylactic treatments prior to the development of spontaneous seizures. The ideal experimental design would conclusively determine whether a therapeutic agent or a target can prevent or reduce the development of unprovoked spontaneous seizures (*i.e.* PTE). The therapeutic time window for certain drugs is narrow and needs to be explored for each potential therapy. Taken together, treatment trials in animal models have identified promising biomarkers and therapeutic targets, but there is a need for better models to screen posttraumatic treatments.

FIG. 11.5, CONT'D   TBI treated with the small-molecule Minozac (TBI-Mzc-ECS), or sham procedure (Sham-ECS; bars indicate median seizure score ± interquartile range). The seizure score was significantly increased in mice subjected to TBI prior to ECS compared to sham controls. Statistical significances between the groups: $P < .05$ (Kruskal-Wallis test). This increase in seizure susceptibility after TBI was prevented by treatment at 3 and 6 h with Mzc (Sham-ECS versus TBI-Mzc-ECS, not significant; $n = 10–12$ per group; TBI, traumatic brain injury). *(Reproduced with permission from Chrzaszcz M, et al. Minozac treatment prevents increased seizure susceptibility in a mouse "two-hit" model of closed skull traumatic brain injury and electroconvulsive shock-induced seizures. J Neurotrauma 2010;27(7):1283–295.)*

References

[1] Cendes F, et al. Neuroimaging of epilepsy. Handb Clin Neurol 2016;136:985–1014.

[2] Amyot F, et al. A review of the effectiveness of neuroimaging modalities for the detection of traumatic brain injury. J Neurotrauma 2015;32(22):1693–721.

[3] Shultz SR, et al. Can structural or functional changes following traumatic brain injury in the rat predict epileptic outcome? Epilepsia 2013;54(7):1240–50.

[4] Di Sapia R, et al. In-depth characterization of a mouse model of post-traumatic epilepsy for biomarker and drug discovery. Acta Neuropathol Commun 2021;9(1):76.

[5] Manninen E, et al. Acute thalamic damage as a prognostic biomarker for post-traumatic epileptogenesis. Epilepsia 2021;62(8):1852–64.

[6] Taupin V, et al. Increase in IL-6, IL-1 and TNF levels in rat brain following traumatic lesion. Influence of pre- and post-traumatic treatment with Ro5 4864, a peripheral-type (p site) benzodiazepine ligand. J Neuroimmunol 1993;42(2):177–85.

[7] Diamond ML, et al. IL-1beta associations with posttraumatic epilepsy development: a genetics and biomarker cohort study. Epilepsia 2014;55(7):1109–19.

[8] Semple BD, et al. Interleukin-1 receptor in seizure susceptibility after traumatic injury to the pediatric brain. J Neurosci 2017;37(33):7864–77.

[9] Pijet B, et al. Elevation of MMP-9 levels promotes epileptogenesis after traumatic brain injury. Mol Neurobiol 2018;55(12):9294–306.

[10] Suehiro E, et al. Increased matrix metalloproteinase-9 in blood in association with activation of interleukin-6 after traumatic brain injury: influence of hypothermic therapy. J Neurotrauma 2004;21(12):1706–11.

[11] Lapinlampi N, et al. Postinjury weight rather than cognitive or behavioral impairment predicts development of posttraumatic epilepsy after lateral fluid-percussion injury in rats. Epilepsia 2020;61(9):2035–52.

[12] Fukudo S, et al. Evidence-based clinical practice guidelines for irritable bowel syndrome 2020. J Gastroenterol 2021;56(3):193–217.

[13] De Leo S, Lee SY, Braverman LE. Hyperthyroidism. Lancet 2016;388(10047):906–18.

[14] Jacobs J, et al. High-frequency oscillations (HFOs) in clinical epilepsy. Prog Neurobiol 2012;98(3):302–15.

[15] Bragin A, et al. Pathologic electrographic changes after experimental traumatic brain injury. Epilepsia 2016;57(5):735–45.

[16] Li L, et al. Spatial and temporal profile of high-frequency oscillations in posttraumatic epileptogenesis. Neurobiol Dis 2021;161, 105544.

[17] Li Q, et al. Baicalein exerts neuroprotective effects in FeCl3-induced posttraumatic epileptic seizures via suppressing ferroptosis. Front Pharmacol 2019;10:638.

[18] Eastman CL, et al. Therapeutic effects of time-limited treatment with brivaracetam on posttraumatic epilepsy after fluid percussion injury in the rat. J Pharmacol Exp Ther 2021;379(3):310–23.

[19] Goodrich GS, et al. Ceftriaxone treatment after traumatic brain injury restores expression of the glutamate transporter, GLT-1, reduces regional gliosis, and reduces post-traumatic seizures in the rat. J Neurotrauma 2013;30(16):1434–41.

[20] Guo D, et al. Rapamycin attenuates the development of posttraumatic epilepsy in a mouse model of traumatic brain injury. PLoS One 2013;8(5), e64078.

[21] Liu SJ, et al. Sodium selenate retards epileptogenesis in acquired epilepsy models reversing changes in protein phosphatase 2A and hyperphosphorylated tau. Brain 2016;139(Pt 7):1919–38.

[22] Echegoyen J, et al. Single application of a CB1 receptor antagonist rapidly following head injury prevents long-term hyperexcitability in a rat model. Epilepsy Res 2009;85(1):123–7.

[23] Nissinen J, et al. Disease-modifying effect of atipamezole in a model of post-traumatic epilepsy. Epilepsy Res 2017;136:18–34.

[24] Chrzaszcz M, et al. Minozac treatment prevents increased seizure susceptibility in a mouse "two-hit" model of closed skull traumatic brain injury and electroconvulsive shock-induced seizures. J Neurotrauma 2010;27(7):1283–95.

[25] Ping X, et al. Blocking receptor for advanced glycation end products (RAGE) or toll-like receptor 4 (TLR4) prevents posttraumatic epileptogenesis in mice. Epilepsia 2021;62(12):3105–16.

[26] Dixon SJ, et al. Ferroptosis: an iron-dependent form of nonapoptotic cell death. Cell 2012;149(5):1060–72.

[27] Srivastava NK, et al. Altered lipid metabolism in post-traumatic epileptic rat model: one proposed pathway. Mol Biol Rep 2019;46(2):1757–73.

[28] Khaleghi F, Nemec II EC. Brivaracetam (Briviact): a novel adjunctive therapy for partial-onset seizures. P T 2017;42(2):92–6.

[29] Ling DSF, Yang L, Goodman JH. Brivaracetam prevents the development of epileptiform activity when administered early after cortical neurotrauma in rats. Epilepsia 2022;63:992–1002.

[30] Rothstein JD, et al. Beta-lactam antibiotics offer neuroprotection by increasing glutamate transporter expression. Nature 2005;433(7021):73–7.

[31] Melzer N, et al. A β-lactam antibiotic dampens excitotoxic inflammatory CNS damage in a mouse model of multiple sclerosis. PLoS One 2008;3(9), e3149.

[32] Lee SG, et al. Mechanism of ceftriaxone induction of excitatory amino acid transporter-2 expression and glutamate uptake in primary human astrocytes. J Biol Chem 2008;283(19):13116–23.

[33] Piao CS, et al. Depression following traumatic brain injury in mice is associated with down-regulation of hippocampal astrocyte glutamate transporters by thrombin. J Cereb Blood Flow Metab 2019;39(1):58–73.

[34] Peterson AR, Binder DK. Post-translational regulation of GLT-1 in neurological diseases and its potential as an effective therapeutic target. Front Mol Neurosci 2019;12(164).

[35] Griffin WC, et al. Effects of ceftriaxone on ethanol drinking and GLT-1 expression in ethanol dependence and relapse drinking. Alcohol 2021;92:1–9.

[36] Bockaert J, Marin P. mTOR in brain physiology and pathologies. Physiol Rev 2015;95(4):1157–87.

[37] Meng XF, et al. Role of the mTOR signaling pathway in epilepsy. J Neurol Sci 2013;332(1–2):4–15.

[38] Barbier P, et al. Role of tau as a microtubule-associated protein: structural and functional aspects. Front Aging Neurosci 2019;11:204.

[39] Thom M, et al. Neurofibrillary tangle pathology and Braak staging in chronic epilepsy in relation to traumatic brain injury and hippocampal sclerosis: a post-mortem study. Brain 2011;134(Pt 10):2969–81.

[40] Machado RA, et al. Reelin, tau phosphorylation and psychiatric complications in patients with hippocampal sclerosis and structural abnormalities in temporal lobe epilepsy. Epilepsy Behav 2019;96:192–9.

[41] Puvenna V, et al. Is phosphorylated tau unique to chronic traumatic encephalopathy? Phosphory-lated tau in epileptic brain and chronic traumatic encephalopathy. Brain Res 2016;1630:225–40.

[42] Shultz SR, et al. Sodium selenate reduces hyperphosphorylated tau and improves outcomes after traumatic brain injury. Brain 2015;138(Pt 5):1297–313.

[43] Xu Y, et al. Structure of a protein phosphatase 2A holoenzyme: insights into B55-mediated tau dephosphorylation. Mol Cell 2008;31(6):873–85.

[44] Ludanyi A, et al. Downregulation of the CB1 cannabinoid receptor and related molecu-lar elements of the endocannabinoid system in epileptic human hippocampus. J Neurosci 2008;28(12):2976–90.

[45] Monory K, et al. The endocannabinoid system controls key epileptogenic circuits in the hip-pocampus. Neuron 2006;51(4):455–66.

[46] Chen K, et al. Prevention of plasticity of endocannabinoid signaling inhibits persistent limbic hyperexcitability caused by developmental seizures. J Neurosci 2007;27(1):46–58.

[47] Pitkanen A, et al. Atipamezole, an alpha(2)-adrenoceptor antagonist, has disease modifying effects on epileptogenesis in rats. Epilepsy Res 2004;61(1–3):119–40.

[48] Halonen T, et al. Alpha 2-adrenoceptor agonist, dexmedetomidine, protects against kainic acid-induced convulsions and neuronal damage. Brain Res 1995;693(1–2):217–24.

[49] Lloyd E, et al. Suppression of acute proinflammatory cytokine and chemokine upregulation by post-injury administration of a novel small molecule improves long-term neurologic outcome in a mouse model of traumatic brain injury. J Neuroinflammation 2008;5:28.

[50] Maroso M, et al. Toll-like receptor 4 and high-mobility group box-1 are involved in ictogen-esis and can be targeted to reduce seizures. Nat Med 2010;16(4):413–9.

[51] Laird MD, et al. High mobility group box protein-1 promotes cerebral edema after traumatic brain injury via activation of toll-like receptor 4. Glia 2014;62(1):26–38.

[52] Paudel YN, et al. HMGB1: a common biomarker and potential target for TBI, neuroinflamma-tion, epilepsy, and cognitive dysfunction. Front Neurosci 2018;12:628.

Chapter 12

Therapeutic targets and future directions

Overview

In this book, we have considered the history (Chapter 1), epidemiology (Chapter 2), and neuropathology (Chapter 3) of posttraumatic epilepsy (PTE); clinical trials of antiepileptogenic agents (Chapter 4); the role of surgical treatment (Chapter 5); and data from animal models of traumatic brain injury (TBI) including potential mechanisms, biomarkers, and treatment trials (Chapters 6–11). Despite all of the work to date, the mechanism(s) underlying posttraumatic epileptogenesis remain unclear, and there is no proven antiepileptogenic agent to prevent PTE after TBI. In this chapter, we outline promising therapeutic targets and discuss suggested future directions for PTE research.

Potential therapeutic targets

To date, clinical trials of agents to prevent PTE have utilized existing antiepileptic drugs (AEDs), but while these have been effective at preventing early seizures after TBI, there has been no demonstrated efficacy on preventing the epileptogenic process leading to late posttraumatic seizures (*i.e.* PTE). Thus, new therapeutic targets should be based on more complete understanding of mechanisms of epileptogenesis after brain injury. While there are many potential targets, here we highlight two categories: inflammation and astrocyte targets.

Inflammation targets

Altering the inflammatory response after TBI holds potential to also alter the likelihood of transition to PTE (Chapter 10). Multiple targets have been considered. The HMGB1 (high-mobility group box protein 1) inhibitor glycyrrhizin reduces microglial activation after TBI and decreases spontaneous seizures [1–3]. Inhibition of RAGE (receptor for advanced glycation end products) or TLR4 (Toll-like receptor 4) after undercut injury reduces astrogliosis and decreases seizure susceptibility [4]. IL-1β (interleukin-1 beta) inhibition reduces neuronal loss, reduces astrogliosis, and decreases seizure susceptibility [5–7]. IL-10 (interleukin-10, an anti-inflammatory cytokine) infusion reduces

Posttraumatic Epilepsy. https://doi.org/10.1016/B978-0-323-90099-7.00014-9

epileptiform activity after TBI [8,9]. Inhibition of the pro-inflammatory cytokine tumor necrosis factor-alpha (TNF-α) improves neurological outcome and reduces ictal discharges [10,11]. Inhibition of macrophage migration inhibitory factor (MIF) reduces astrogliosis and peripheral lymphocyte activation following TBI [12]. Inhibition of TLR decreases seizure susceptibility and reduces TNF-α levels after TBI [13]. Inhibition of transforming growth factor-beta (TGF-β) with losartan decreases seizure susceptibility in an albumin-induced model of epilepsy [14].

While all of the above studies suggest that various cytokine pathways influence seizure susceptibility, to date there are no long-term studies of any of the above mechanisms in a PTE model with an outcome of decreasing late *spontaneous recurrent seizures* (PTE). Such studies are urgently needed. In addition, it may be of interest to take a different approach to influencing neuroinflammatory pathways that goes beyond a "single cytokine modulation" strategy. For example, driving M2-like polarization in macrophages could possibly be used as a strategy to prevent PTE [15]. Stat6 (signal transducer and activator of transcription 6) has been proposed to drive macrophage M2 polarization. Inhibition of Stat6 acetylation promotes M2 polarization in macrophages [16]. Hypothetically, M2 polarization would be a broader and thus potentially more efficacious therapeutic technique than "single cytokine modulation."

Astrocyte targets

Astrocytes play an established role in removal of glutamate at synapses and the sequestration and redistribution of K^+ and H_2O during neural activity [17,18]. It is becoming increasingly clear that changes in astrocyte channels, transporters, and metabolism play a direct role in seizure susceptibility and the development of epilepsy [17,19–25]. Stimulation of astrocytes leads to prolonged neuronal depolarization and epileptiform discharges [24]. Astrocytes release neuroactive molecules and modulate synaptic transmission through modifications in channels, gap junctions, receptors, and transporters [17,19,24,26–31]. Furthermore, striking changes in astrocyte form and function occur in epilepsy. Astrocytes adopt reactive morphology [20,32], become uncoupled [33], and lose domain organization [34] in epileptic tissue. These and other changes such as changes in the expression of various astrocytic enzymes, such as adenosine kinase [35] and glutamine synthetase [36], astroglial proliferation, dysregulation of water and ion channel and glutamate transporter expression [17,37,38], alterations in secretion of neuroactive molecules, and increased activation of inflammatory pathways [20,23,32,39–42], may all contribute to hyperexcitability and epileptogenesis [43].

Glutamate transporters

Glutamate transporters are expressed by several central nervous system (CNS) cell types, but astrocytes are primarily responsible for glutamate uptake. Studies using mice with deletion [44] or antisense oligonucleotide-mediated inhibition of synthesis [45] of the astroglial transporter GLT-1 (glutamate transporter-1, also named EAAT2) revealed that this subtype is responsible for the bulk of extracellular glutamate clearance in the CNS [46]. Several studies have suggested an involvement of glutamate transporters in seizure development. GLT-1 knockout in mice caused spontaneous seizures and hippocampal pathology resembling alterations in patients with temporal lobe epilepsy (TLE) with mesial temporal sclerosis (MTS) [44]. A more recent follow-up paper by the same group using region-specific GLT-1 knockout mice confirmed spontaneous seizures when GLT-1 was deleted from forebrain astrocytes [47].

What is the evidence for alteration in astrocyte glutamate transporters in human epilepsy specimens and in animal models? Decreased GLT-1 immunoreactivity has been reported in the sclerotic human hippocampus, although GLAST (glutamate aspartate transporter, also named EAAT1) immunoreactivity was reported as unchanged [48] or decreased [49]. These findings support the hypothesis that reduced or dysfunctional glial glutamate transporters in the hippocampus may trigger spontaneous seizures in patients [50]. A study in the mouse intrahippocampal kainic acid (IHKA) model found a significant initial increase in dorsal hippocampal GLT-1 immunoreactivity and protein levels 1 day after status epilepticus followed by a marked downregulation at 4 and 7 days after status epilepticus, a time period during which spontaneous seizures arise in this model [37]. Interestingly, GLT-1 immunoreactivity and synaptosomal protein levels were significantly downregulated at 7 days post-IHKA in the ipsilateral hippocampus [51]. Therefore, early GLT-1 dysregulation may precede spontaneous seizures and thus contribute to epileptogenesis.

The above studies were done in models of temporal lobe epilepsy with hippocampal sclerosis. Similar evidence for glutamate transporter dysregulation has been observed following TBI in parallel to a decrease in glutamate clearance which could contribute to the development of epilepsy [52–54]. Treating rats with ceftriaxone daily post-TBI restores GLT-1 expression in the lesioned cortex compared to vehicle-treated animals following fluid percussion injury (FPI) and reduces posttraumatic seizures [55]. In a model of repeated diffuse TBI, mice that developed PTE had significantly more GLT-1 downregulation than mice that did not develop PTE [53]. Thus, GLT-1 downregulation appears to contribute to PTE in these studies. Viral upregulation of GLT-1 has been found to be neuroprotective and antiepileptogenic in the intrahippocampal kainic acid model of epilepsy [56]. Therefore, GLT-1 upregulation appears to be a promising potential strategy to prevent PTE after TBI and should be further studied.

Aquaporin-4

The aquaporins (AQPs) are a family of membrane proteins that function as "water channels" in many cell types and tissues in which fluid transport is crucial [57]. Aquaporin-4 (AQP4) is expressed ubiquitously by glial cells, especially at specialized membrane domains including astroglial endfeet in contact with blood vessels and astrocyte membranes that ensheathe glutamatergic synapses. Mice deficient in AQP4 have markedly decreased accumulation of brain water (cerebral edema) following water intoxication and focal cerebral ischemia [58] and impaired clearance of brain water in models of vasogenic edema [59], suggesting a functional role for AQP4 in brain water transport. In addition, AQP4 knockout mice have remarkably impaired K^+ clearance and prolonged seizures in response to *in vivo* hippocampal stimulation [60]. These data suggest that AQP4 downregulation may trigger hyperexcitability.

Alteration in the expression and subcellular localization of AQP4 has been described in sclerotic hippocampi obtained from patients with MTS. Using immunohistochemistry, rt-PCR, and gene chip analysis, Lee *et al.* demonstrated an overall increase in AQP4 expression in sclerotic hippocampi [61]. However, using quantitative immunogold electron microscopy, the same group found mislocalization of AQP4 in the human epileptic hippocampus, with reduction in perivascular membrane expression [62]. The authors hypothesized that the loss of perivascular AQP4 perturbs water flux, impairs K^+ buffering, and results in an increased propensity for seizures.

Subsequently, very similar AQP4 dysregulation has been confirmed in animal models of epilepsy. In particular, downregulation and/or mislocalization of AQP4 occur during the early epileptogenic phase in the rat pilocarpine [63,64], rat kainic acid [65], and mouse kainic acid [37,38] models of epilepsy. Similar evidence for aquaporin dysregulation has recently been observed following TBI. In a mouse model of controlled cortical impact (CCI), a significant increase in AQP4 in the ipsilateral frontal cortex and hippocampus of mice that developed PTE compared to those that did not develop PTE was found; but interestingly, AQP4 was also found to be mislocalized away from the perivascular endfeet and toward the neuropil in mice that developed PTE [66], very reminiscent of the original findings in human temporal lobe epilepsy [62]. Thus, these recent PTE data coincide with AQP4 dysregulation in other models of epilepsy and in human epilepsy [17,25,65,67]. In addition, upregulation of AQP4 improves blood-brain barrier integrity and perihematomal edema following intracerebral hemorrhage [68]. Thus, restoration of AQP4 homeostasis and localization may serve to restore water and potassium homeostasis and limit posttraumatic hyperexcitability. Recent efficacy in treatment of CNS edema has been found by targeting the mechanism of calmodulin-mediated cell-surface localization of AQP4: remarkably, inhibition of calmodulin with the drug trifluoperazine inhibited AQP4 mislocalization, ablated CNS edema, and improved functional recovery after spinal cord injury [69]. It is conceivable that a similar approach to modulation of AQP4 may be therapeutic in preventing AQP4 mislocalization after TBI and thereby inhibiting PTE development.

Other astrocyte targets

While not addressed yet in PTE studies, other astrocyte targets have arisen as contributing to other forms of epilepsy. These include Kir4.1 (inwardly rectifying

K^+ channel) [70–72], glutamine synthetase [73,74], adenosine [75,76], and gap junctional coupling [33,71,72]. Recently, both Kir4.1 and glutamine synthetase were found to be downregulated in a model of repeated diffuse TBI [53]. Clearly, these molecules should be fully evaluated in the appropriate PTE animal models to determine the best possible astrocyte targets for antiepileptogenic strategies after TBI.

Future directions for preclinical posttraumatic epilepsy research

We submit the following points as key future directions for preclinical PTE research.

1. Optimize PTE animal models.
   Of critical importance is the use of appropriate animal models of PTE. The most important criteria for these models are that they not only are well-accepted models of TBI *but also* that they recapitulate the delayed onset of late spontaneous recurrent seizures (SRS, *i.e.* PTE). Many earlier studies (Chapter 7) have assessed seizure *susceptibility* at various time points following TBI using chemoconvulsant (*e.g.* pentylenetetrazole (PTZ) or kainic acid) threshold testing. However, such chemoconvulsant thresholds are not spontaneous seizures, and thus results from such studies cannot be generalized into implications for PTE pathogenesis or treatment.
   Earlier papers with FPI and CCI models indicated quite low yield of PTE [77]. However, more recent papers have used more severe CCI to attain adequate yield of mice developing PTE after CCI. For example, Szu *et al.* used a 2-mm flat impactor tip at a velocity of 5 m/s, a depth of 1 mm, and a contact time of 200 ms to generate a moderate-severe TBI, performed long-term video-electroencephalography (EEG) monitoring, and found a PTE yield of 20% at 30 days and 27% at 60 days [66]. Di Sapia *et al.* induced CCI using a 3-mm-diameter rigid impactor at an impactor velocity of 5 m/s and deformation depth of 2 mm, resulting in severe injury. In this study, PTE yield was 45% at 3.5 months and 58% at 5 months; however, mortality was high (35%) [78].
   In addition to achieving adequate PTE yield from the animal model, appropriate long-term video-EEG monitoring must be performed to accurately identify which mice develop seizures and which do not after TBI. Long-term video-EEG monitoring can be quite time-intensive to analyze. Thus, the development of validated automated seizure detection software and its application to long-term EEG recordings is of key importance [56,79]. One such MATLAB algorithm with a customized graphical user interface (GUI) and user-defined selection of seizure parameters is freely accessible online at the following public repository: https://github.com/eplab1745/ESA_Extended [56].
   Using such software, screening of long-term EEG recordings for positive electrophysiological seizures can then be performed, and each individual

seizure can be analyzed for behavioral changes (seizure score) timed to the electrophysiological change. Importantly, such analysis should be done blinded to treatment, and interobserver reliability of seizure scoring within the research team should be carefully documented. It is also important to exclude poor-quality EEG recordings, and therefore, each EEG research team should carefully document artifact rejection and only analyze artifact-free EEG recordings. Finally, clear seizure outcome measures should be recorded. These include seizure numbers/frequency, seizure duration, total seizure time (frequency × duration), and behavioral seizure scores with the Racine scale [80]. Finally, to the extent that biomarkers (such as EEG biomarkers, see below) can be *incorporated* into the study design, then a great deal more useful data can emanate from these intensive long-term studies beyond just seizure outcomes.

2. Conduct detailed electrophysiological analyses of the PTE *vs.* non-PTE brain.

In vivo

There may be many events occurring in the "PTE brain" other than just seizures. In other words, detailed modern electrophysiological analysis of long-term high-quality EEG recordings from brains that develop PTE after TBI *vs.* those that do not may yield PTE-specific EEG biomarkers. Such EEG biomarkers of PTE could have both prognostic and therapeutic significance. For example, high-frequency oscillations (HFOs) have been found to serve as a biomarker for epilepsy [81,82]. In the lateral fluid percussion injury (LFPI) model, early predictors of PTE development noted are the emergence of pathological HFOs (100–600 Hz) and repetitive HFOs with spikes (rHFOSs) [83,84]. Other derived EEG parameters may be quite interesting to assess as potential biomarkers of the "early epileptogenic network" in PTE. Some EEG parameters that are available to apply to PTE include power spectral density (PSD) analysis [85], connectivity analyses [86,87], phase coherence, and cross-frequency amplitude coupling [86]. Connectivity analyses between electrodes located in the perilesional zone and distant electrodes may indicate an altered interplay of connectivity in mice that develop PTE *vs.* mice that do not after TBI. Validation of such EEG biomarkers for PTE would then enable treatment/antiepileptogenesis trials to have as outcomes not only the final effect on PTE itself but also intermediate effects on EEG biomarkers of PTE.

Ex vivo

Similarly, *ex vivo* physiological studies of slices from PTE brains *vs.* post-TBI brains that did not develop PTE should be undertaken to understand the specific physiological underpinnings of PTE. Physiological analyses should ideally be done both in perilesional areas (*e.g.* the cortex around a CCI lesion) and in distant areas that may undergo posttraumatic epileptogenesis (*e.g.* hippocampus). Ideally, *ex vivo* physiology studies should engage both potential neuronal and astrocytic mechanisms.

3. Examine the loci of PTE development in the brain.

Despite the clinical significance of PTE, the locus of where PTE develops relative to the site of head injury and thus the anatomy of development of PTE in distributed brain networks are not well understood. In particular, whether PTE develops from seizure foci originating in the perilesional cortex (around the impact site) *vs.* distributed networks that become hyperexcitable in distant anatomical structures (such as the hippocampus) has not been determined. Thus, a key "knowledge gap" in the understanding of PTE is defining the exact anatomic locus of PTE development relative to the site(s) of brain injury, and which cellular and molecular changes occur uniquely in that locus that underlie PTE development [88].

One technology that could be applied to PTE research is multielectrode array (MEA) technology. MEA studies allow for simultaneous multisite recordings over the surface of the brain [85,87], and, combined with depth electrode implantation, could be employed to determine PTE site(s) of onset and spread after injury with much greater anatomic specificity. For example, MEA implemented with depth electrode implantation in the hippocampus could enable determination of perilesional *vs.* hippocampal seizure onset. These studies could enable the definition of the anatomic basis for PTE onset in the CCI model for the first time. In addition, MEA technology enables detailed connectivity analyses.

4. Conduct cellular/molecular analyses of PTE *vs.* non-PTE brains.

Clearly needed are studies that determine which cellular and molecular changes are associated with PTE onset. The presence of molecular changes in mice with PTE that are not observed in nonepileptic post-TBI mice is supported by the recent demonstration of dysregulation and mislocalization of AQP4 specifically in mice with PTE [66]. These data raise the possibility that alterations in astrocytic transporter localization herald emergence of the putative seizure focus. Furthermore, in light of the proposed association between AQP4 and the astrocytic glutamate transporter GLT-1 [89], one would expect GLT-1 reduction and mislocalization to parallel that of AQP4 in the seizure focus [51,66,90]. Indeed, previous studies have found reduction in glutamate clearance in the perilesional cortex after CCI [91], which could impair excitation:inhibition (E:I) balance. One recent study found more "GLT-1 deleted" areas in mice that developed PTE after repeated diffuse TBI than those that did not [53], thus correlating GLT-1 loss to PTE onset. Interestingly, these types of studies may help to rule out other astrocyte molecular candidates. For example, in the Szu *et al.* study, unlike for AQP4, there was no correlation between Kir4.1 levels or distribution and PTE onset [66].

Whatever the final findings, the key strategy is to evaluate cellular and molecular changes that are *specific* to the animals developing PTE compared to those subjected to the same injury (whether CCI or FPI, *etc.*) that do not develop PTE. This requires a combination of careful and detailed electrophysiological analysis to clearly define the PTE *vs.* non-PTE subgroups after TBI, and then conducting careful cellular/molecular analysis to understand what is different in PTE brains.

5. Examine treatment windows.

Treatment trials should separately analyze effects of a given agent on neuroprotection after TBI and epileptogenesis after TBI. If an agent were given *early* after TBI, it may possibly be early enough to help prevent secondary injury from the TBI and thus have a neuroprotective effect. Presumably, if given in a later time window after injury, the same agent may not have any neuroprotective effect on the initial TBI as that initial TBI and secondary injury would have already taken effect (and therefore too late to "improve" histology), but the process of epileptogenesis after TBI may still be underway and there still may be a therapeutic "window" for antiepileptogenic intervention.

This formulation may help to predict the outcome of various interventions in terms of expected efficacy in specific time windows. *Late* engagement of cytokine mechanisms may be ineffective if the cytokine modulation window of efficacy is *early* after TBI. This may be expected if inflammatory changes all occur within several days of the initial TBI (at least acute inflammatory changes). Thus, intervening with cytokine-modulating drugs may be most effective early after injury. In contrast, *late* engagement of long-term glial/astrocyte changes such as alteration in AQP4 localization or GLT-1 perisynaptic localization may be more amenable to a treatment that is delayed after the initial injury. In other words, 1 month after injury, it still may be quite helpful to upregulate GLT-1 around synapses to clamp glutamate levels within a subseizure range, whereas modulating cytokines 1 month after injury may be "too little, too late" to prevent or modulate the epileptogenic process.

6. Evaluate various "levels" of epileptogenesis.

Treatment trials should *also* evaluate the effect on epileptogenesis in the *perilesional zone* versus what one might call *distal epileptogenesis*. If a given agent fails to prevent perilesional epileptogenesis but does prevent distal epileptogenesis, this still may be of significant therapeutic value in preventing seizure spread throughout the brain. Such a therapeutic agent would facilitate confining PTE to "local PTE" and not "generalized PTE." To analyze this, multisite multielectrode recordings will be useful with electrodes covering both the perilesional area and the distant sites (*e.g.* hippocampus) to separately assess the timing and extent of epileptogenesis in the perilesional area *vs.* distant sites. Specific metrics of "spreading seizures" as have been described [92] can then be characterized. An agent given too late to disrupt perilesional epileptogenesis but that still has efficacy against distal epileptogenesis may still have therapeutic value.

Summary

Careful electrophysiological, cellular, and molecular phenotyping of PTE (as compared to TBI without PTE) will enable more precise and selective therapies to alter or inhibit cellular and molecular and physiological changes that underlie PTE. Ultimately, the above studies should determine the neural circuit underlying PTE, whether this involves alterations in connectivity/sprouting of new synapses in perilesional *vs.* distant areas, alteration of existing synapses, alteration of inflammatory milieu, alteration of astrocyte molecules and metabolism, altered nonsynaptic mechanisms, or some combination of the above. The main goal of this work is to elucidate the nature of Penfield's "silent period of strange ripening" resulting in posttraumatic epileptogenesis [93]. Mechanism-based understanding of PTE should lead to mechanism-based therapeutics, tailored to specific possible windows of intervention after TBI.

References

[1] Kan M, et al. Circulating high mobility group box-1 and toll-like receptor 4 expressions increase the risk and severity of epilepsy. Braz J Med Biol Res 2019;52(7), e7374.

[2] Webster KM, et al. Targeting high-mobility group box protein 1 (HMGB1) in pediatric traumatic brain injury: chronic neuroinflammatory, behavioral, and epileptogenic consequences. Exp Neurol 2019;320, 112979.

[3] Webster KM, et al. Inflammation in epileptogenesis after traumatic brain injury. J Neuroinflammation 2017;14(1):10.

[4] Ping X, et al. Blocking receptor for advanced glycation end products (RAGE) or toll-like receptor 4 (TLR4) prevents posttraumatic epileptogenesis in mice. Epilepsia 2021;62(12):3105–16.

[5] Lu KT, et al. Effect of interleukin-1 on traumatic brain injury-induced damage to hippocampal neurons. J Neurotrauma 2005;22(8):885–95.

[6] Semple BD, et al. Interleukin-1 receptor in seizure susceptibility after traumatic injury to the pediatric brain. J Neurosci 2017;37(33):7864–77.

[7] Zou H, et al. Neuroprotective, neuroplastic, and neurobehavioral effects of daily treatment with levetiracetam in experimental traumatic brain injury. Neurorehabil Neural Repair 2013;27(9):878–88.

[8] Knoblach SM, Faden AI. Interleukin-10 improves outcome and alters proinflammatory cytokine expression after experimental traumatic brain injury. Exp Neurol 1998;153(1):143–51.

[9] Levin SG, Godukhin OV. Protective effects of interleukin-10 on the development of epileptiform activity evoked by transient episodes of hypoxia in rat hippocampal slices. Neurosci Behav Physiol 2007;37(5):467–70.

[10] Chio CC, et al. Etanercept attenuates traumatic brain injury in rats by reducing early microglial expression of tumor necrosis factor-alpha. BMC Neurosci 2013;14:33.

[11] Chong SA, et al. Intrinsic inflammation is a potential anti-epileptogenic target in the organotypic hippocampal slice model. Neurotherapeutics 2018;15(2):470–88.

[12] Newell-Rogers MK, et al. Antagonism of macrophage migration inhibitory factor (MIF) after traumatic brain injury ameliorates astrocytosis and peripheral lymphocyte activation and expansion. Int J Mol Sci 2020;21(20).

[13] Hesam S, et al. Monophosphoryl lipid A and Pam3Cys prevent the increase in seizure susceptibility and epileptogenesis in rats undergoing traumatic brain injury. Neurochem Res 2018;43(10):1978–85.

[14] Bar-Klein G, et al. Losartan prevents acquired epilepsy via TGF-beta signaling suppression. Ann Neurol 2014;75(6):864–75.

[15] Therajaran P, et al. Microglial polarization in posttraumatic epilepsy: potential mechanism and treatment opportunity. Epilepsia 2020;61(2):203–15.

[16] Yu T, et al. Modulation of M2 macrophage polarization by the crosstalk between Stat6 and Trim24. Nat Commun 2019;10(1):4353.

[17] Binder DK, Nagelhus EA, Ottersen OP. Aquaporin-4 and epilepsy. Glia 2012;60(8):1203–14.

[18] Ransom B, Behar T, Nedergaard M. New roles for astrocytes (stars at last). Trends Neurosci 2003;26:520–2.

[19] Binder DK, Steinhäuser C. Functional changes in astroglial cells in epilepsy. Glia 2006;54:358–68.

[20] Clasadonte J, Haydon PG. Astrocytes and epilepsy. In: Noebles JL, Avoli M, Rogawski MA, Olsen RW, Delgado-Escueta AV, editors. Jasper's basic mechanisms of the epilepsies; 2012. p. 19.

[21] Friedman A, Kaufer D, Heinemann U. Blood-brain barrier breakdown-inducing astrocytic transformation: novel targets for the prevention of epilepsy. Epilepsy Res 2009;85:142–9.

[22] Seifert G, Carmignoto G, Steinhäuser C. Astrocyte dysfunction in epilepsy. Brain Res Rev 2010;63:212–21.

[23] Seifert G, Schilling K, Steinhäuser C. Astrocyte dysfunction in neurological disorders: a molecular perspective. Nat Rev Neurosci 2006;7(3):194–206.

[24] Tian G, et al. An astrocytic basis of epilepsy. Nat Med 2005;11(9):973–81.

[25] Binder DK, Steinhäuser C. Astrocytes and epilepsy. Neurochem Res 2021;46(10):2687–95.

[26] Beenhakker MP, Huguenard JR. Astrocytes as gatekeepers of GABAB receptor function. J Neurosci 2010;30(45):15262–76.

[27] Halassa MM, Fellin T, Haydon PG. The tripartite synapse: roles for gliotransmission in health and disease. Trends Mol Med 2007;13(2):54–63.

[28] Rouach N, et al. Astroglial metabolic networks sustain hippocampal synaptic transmission. Science 2008;322(5907):1551–5.

[29] Santello M, Bezzi P, Volterra A. TNF-alpha controls glutamatergic gliotransmission in the hippocampal dentate gyrus. Neuron 2011;69(5):988–1001.

[30] Volterra A, Steinhäuser C. Glial modulation of synaptic transmission in the hippocampus. Glia 2004;47(3):249–57.

[31] Wang F, et al. Astrocytes modulate neural network activity by Ca^{2+}-dependent uptake of extracellular K^+. Sci Signal 2012;5(218):ra26.

[32] Heinemann U, et al. Alterations of glial cell function in temporal lobe epilepsy. Epilepsia 2000;41(Suppl 6):S185–9.

[33] Bedner P, et al. Astrocyte uncoupling as a cause of human temporal lobe epilepsy. Brain 2015;138(Pt 5):1208–22.

[34] Oberheim NA, et al. Loss of astrocytic domain organization in the epileptic brain. J Neurosci 2008;28(13):3264–76.

[35] Aronica E, et al. Upregulation of adenosine kinase in astrocytes in experimental and human temporal lobe epilepsy. Epilepsia 2011;52(9):1645–55.

[36] Coulter DA, Eid T. Astrocytic regulation of glutamate homeostasis in epilepsy. Glia 2012;60:1215–26.

[37] Hubbard JA, et al. Regulation of astrocyte glutamate transporter-1 (GLT1) and aquaporin-4 (AQP4) expression in a model of epilepsy. Exp Neurol 2016;283(Pt A):85–96.

[38] Lee DJ, et al. Decreased expression of the glial water channel aquaporin-4 in the intrahippocampal kainic acid model of epileptogenesis. Exp Neurol 2012;235(1):246–55.

[39] de Lanerolle NC, Lee T. New facets of the neuropathology and molecular profile of human temporal lobe epilepsy. Epilepsy Behav 2005;7:190–203.

[40] Steinhäuser C, Seifert G. Glial membrane channels and receptors in epilepsy: impact for generation and spread of seizure activity. Eur J Pharmacol 2002;447(2–3):227–37.

[41] Hinterkeuser S, et al. Astrocytes in the hippocampus of patients with temporal lobe epilepsy display changes in potassium conductances. Eur J Neurosci 2000;12(6):2087–96.

[42] Kivi A, et al. Effects of barium on stimulus-induced rises of $[K^+]_o$ in human epileptic nonsclerotic and sclerotic hippocampal area CA1. Eur J Neurosci 2000;12(6):2039–48.

[43] Hubbard JA, Binder DK. Astrocytes and epilepsy. Elsevier: Academic Press; 2016.

[44] Tanaka K, et al. Epilepsy and exacerbation of brain injury in mice lacking the glutamate transporter GLT-1. Science 1997;276(5319):1699–702.

[45] Rothstein JD, et al. Knockout of glutamate transporters reveals a major role for astroglial transport in excitotoxicity and clearance of glutamate. Neuron 1996;16(3):675–86.

[46] Danbolt NC. Glutamate uptake. Prog Neurobiol 2001;65(1):1–105.

[47] Sugimoto J, et al. Region-specific deletions of the glutamate transporter GLT1 differentially affect seizure activity and neurodegeneration in mice. Glia 2018;66(4):777–88.

[48] Mathern GW, et al. Hippocampal GABA and glutamate transporter immunoreactivity in patients with temporal lobe epilepsy. Neurology 1999;52(3):453–72.

[49] Proper EA, et al. Distribution of glutamate transporters in the hippocampus of patients with pharmaco-resistant temporal lobe epilepsy. Brain 2002;125(Pt 1):32–43.

[50] During MJ, Spencer DD. Extracellular hippocampal glutamate and spontaneous seizure in the conscious human brain. Lancet 1993;341(8861):1607–10.

[51] Peterson AR, Binder DK. Regulation of synaptosomal GLT-1 and GLAST during epileptogenesis. Neuroscience 2019;411:185–201.

[52] Piao CS, et al. Depression following traumatic brain injury in mice is associated with downregulation of hippocampal astrocyte glutamate transporters by thrombin. J Cereb Blood Flow Metab 2019;39(1):58–73.

[53] Shandra O, et al. Repetitive diffuse mild traumatic brain injury causes an atypical astrocyte response and spontaneous recurrent seizures. J Neurosci 2019;39(10):1944–63.

[54] Samuelsson C, et al. Decreased cortical levels of astrocytic glutamate transport protein GLT-1 in a rat model of posttraumatic epilepsy. Neurosci Lett 2000;289(3):185–8.

[55] Goodrich GS, et al. Ceftriaxone treatment after traumatic brain injury restores expression of the glutamate transporter, GLT-1, reduces regional gliosis, and reduces post-traumatic seizures in the rat. J Neurotrauma 2013;30(16):1434–41.

[56] Peterson AR, et al. Targeted overexpression of glutamate transporter-1 reduces seizures and attenuates pathological changes in a mouse model of epilepsy. Neurobiol Dis 2021;157, 105443.

[57] Verkman AS. More than just water channels: unexpected cellular roles of aquaporins. J Cell Sci 2005;118(Pt 15):3225–32.

[58] Manley GT, et al. Aquaporin-4 deletion in mice reduces brain edema after acute water intoxication and ischemic stroke. Nat Med 2000;6(2):159–63.

[59] Papadopoulos MC, et al. Aquaporin-4 facilitates reabsorption of excess fluid in vasogenic brain edema. FASEB J 2004;18(11):1291–3.

[60] Binder DK, et al. Increased seizure duration and slowed potassium kinetics in mice lacking aquaporin-4 water channels. Glia 2006;53:631–6.

[61] Lee TS, et al. Aquaporin-4 is increased in the sclerotic hippocampus in human temporal lobe epilepsy. Acta Neuropathol (Berl) 2004;108(6):493–502.

[62] Eid T, et al. Loss of perivascular aquaporin-4 may underlie deficient water and K^+ homeostasis in the human epileptogenic hippocampus. Proc Natl Acad Sci U S A 2005;102(4):1193–8.

[63] Kim JE, et al. Differential expressions of aquaporin subtypes in astroglia in the hippocampus of chronic epileptic rats. Neuroscience 2009;163(3):781–9.

[64] Kim JE, et al. Astroglial loss and edema formation in the rat piriform cortex and hippocampus following pilocarpine-induced status epilepticus. J Comp Neurol 2010;518(22):4612–28.

[65] Alvestad S, et al. Mislocalization of AQP4 precedes chronic seizures in the kainate model of temporal lobe epilepsy. Epilepsy Res 2013;105(1–2):30–41.

[66] Szu JI, et al. Aquaporin-4 dysregulation in a controlled cortical impact injury model of post-traumatic epilepsy. Neuroscience 2020;428:140–53.

[67] Binder DK. Astrocytes: stars of the sacred disease. Epilepsy Curr 2018;18(3):172–9.

[68] Jeon H, et al. Upregulation of AQP4 improves blood-brain barrier integrity and perihematomal edema following intracerebral hemorrhage. Neurotherapeutics 2021;18(4):2692–706.

[69] Kitchen P, et al. Targeting aquaporin-4 subcellular localization to treat central nervous system edema. Cell 2020;181(4):784–799 e19.

[70] Ivens S, et al. TGF-beta receptor-mediated albumin uptake into astrocytes is involved in neocortical epileptogenesis. Brain 2007;130(Pt 2):535–47.

[71] Bedner P, Steinhäuser C. Altered Kir and gap junction channels in temporal lobe epilepsy. Neurochem Int 2013;63(7):682–7.

[72] Steinhäuser C, Seifert G, Bedner P. Astrocyte dysfunction in temporal lobe epilepsy: K^+ channels and gap junction coupling. Glia 2012;60(8):1192–202.

[73] Eid T, et al. Loss of glutamine synthetase in the human epileptogenic hippocampus: possible mechanism for raised extracellular glutamate in mesial temporal lobe epilepsy. Lancet 2004;363(9402):28–37.

[74] Sandhu MRS, et al. Astroglial glutamine synthetase and the pathogenesis of mesial temporal lobe epilepsy. Front Neurol 2021;12, 665334.

[75] Boison D. Adenosine dysfunction in epilepsy. Glia 2012;60(8):1234–43.

[76] Weltha L, Reemmer J, Boison D. The role of adenosine in epilepsy. Brain Res Bull 2019;151:46–54.

[77] Bolkvadze T, Pitkanen A. Development of post-traumatic epilepsy after controlled cortical impact and lateral fluid-percussion-induced brain injury in the mouse. J Neurotrauma 2012;29(5):789–812.

[78] Di Sapia R, et al. In-depth characterization of a mouse model of post-traumatic epilepsy for biomarker and drug discovery. Acta Neuropathol Commun 2021;9(1):76.

[79] Zeidler Z, et al. Targeting the mouse ventral hippocampus in the intrahippocampal kainic acid model of temporal lobe epilepsy. eNeuro 2018;5(4).

[80] Racine RJ. Modification of seizure activity by electrical stimulation. II Motor seizure. Electroencephalogr Clin Neurophysiol 1972;32(3):281–94.

[81] Ewell LA, et al. The impact of pathological high-frequency oscillations on hippocampal network activity in rats with chronic epilepsy. Elife 2019;8.

[82] Weiss SA, et al. Ictal onset patterns of local field potentials, high frequency oscillations, and unit activity in human mesial temporal lobe epilepsy. Epilepsia 2016;57(1):111–21.

[83] Bragin A, et al. Pathologic electrographic changes after experimental traumatic brain injury. Epilepsia 2016;57(5):735–45.

[84] Li L, et al. Spatial and temporal profile of high-frequency oscillations in posttraumatic epileptogenesis. Neurobiol Dis 2021;161, 105544.

[85] Jonak CR, et al. Multielectrode array analysis of EEG biomarkers in a mouse model of Fragile X Syndrome. Neurobiol Dis 2020;138, 104794.

[86] Wang J, et al. A resting EEG study of neocortical hyperexcitability and altered functional connectivity in fragile X syndrome. J Neurodev Disord 2017;9:11.

[87] Jonak CR, et al. Reusable multielectrode array technique for electroencephalography in awake freely moving mice. Front Integr Neurosci 2018;12:53.

[88] Binder DK, et al. Epilepsy benchmarks area II: prevent epilepsy and its progression. Epilepsy Curr 2020;20(1_suppl):14S–22S.

[89] Wang H, et al. Aquaporin-4 forms a macromolecular complex with glutamate transporter-1 and mu opioid receptor in astrocytes and participates in morphine dependence. J Mol Neurosci 2017;62(1):17–27.

[90] Peterson AR, Binder DK. Astrocyte glutamate uptake and signaling as novel targets for anti-epileptogenic therapy. Front Neurol 2020;11:1006.

[91] Armbruster M, Hanson E, Dulla CG. Glutamate clearance is locally modulated by presynaptic neuronal activity in the cerebral cortex. J Neurosci 2016;36(40):10404–15.

[92] Eastman CL, et al. Therapeutic effects of time-limited treatment with brivaracetam on posttraumatic epilepsy after fluid percussion injury in the rat. J Pharmacol Exp Ther 2021;379(3):310–23.

[93] Penfield W. Introduction (symposium on post-traumatic epilepsy). Epilepsia 1961;2:109–10.

Index

Note: Page numbers followed by *f* indicate figures and *t* indicate tables.

A

Adventitial/nonnervous cells, 47–48
Ammoniacal silver carbonate method, 50
Aquaporin-4 (AQP4), 171–172
  dysregulation, mislocalization of, 117–118,
    117*f*
Aquaporins (AQPs), 129–130
Astrocyte targets, 170–173
  aquaporin-4, 171–172
  glutamate transporters, 170–171
  other astrocyte targets, 172–173
Astrocytic transforming growth factor-beta
    signaling, 130–133
Atipamezole (ATI), 161–163, 162–163*f*

B

Baicalein, 156
Biomarkers
  electrophysiological biomarkers, 155, 156*t*
  imaging biomarkers, 153–154, 154*f*
  postinjury weight loss, 155
  protein biomarkers, 154–155
Blast-induced traumatic brain injury (bTBI), 110
Blood-brain barrier disruption
  chronic dysfunction, 125, 133
  edema, 127
  gadolinium-DTPA (Gd-DTPA), 125
  glial influence on, 129–133
    aquaporins (AQPs), 129–130
    astrocytic transforming growth factor-beta
      signaling, 130–133
    cation-chloride cotransporters, 130
    serum albumin, 130–133, 131*f*
  serum albumin, 120, 122*f*
  tight junctions, 127–129, 128–129*f*
  traumatic brain injury (TBI), 119–126, 121*f*
Brivaracetam, 158

C

Cannabinoid type-1 (CB1) receptor signaling,
    160, 161*f*
Carbamazepine study, 68

Cation-chloride cotransporters, 130
Ceftriaxone, 158
Cellular and molecular changes
  aquaporin-4 dysregulation, mislocalization
    of, 117–118, 117*f*
  mossy fiber sprouting, 115, 116*f*
  reactive astrocytes, 115–116
Central nervous system (CNS),
    43–44
Cerebral cicatrix, 53
Chronic dysfunction, 125, 133
Chronic neuroinflammation, 137
Cicatricial contraction, 78
Cicatrix, 53–56
Civilian injuries, 34–36, 35*t*, 36*f*
Clasmatodendrosis, 54
Clinical heterogeneity, 38–39
Controlled cortical impact (CCI) injury model,
    91–92, 92*f*, 108, 109*f*, 115
Cortical localization, 7–12
  language functions, localization of,
    7–9, 8*f*
  motor functions localization, 9–12, 11*f*
Craniotomy, trephination to, 4–7

D

Dandy-Walker syndrome, 73–74
Discharging lesion, 56

E

Edema, 127
Electroencephalography (EEG), 81–82
Electrocorticography (ECoG), 78, 83
Electrophysiological biomarkers, 155,
    156*t*

F

Feeney model, 93, 93*f*
Fluid percussion injury (FPI), 91, 92*f*, 105,
    106–107*t*, 107*f*
Foerster, Otfrid, 20–24, 22–23*f*
Frontal lobe epilepsy (FLE), 82

G

Gadolinium-DTPA (Gd-DTPA), 125
Glasgow Coma Scale, 63*t*
Glial cells, 138–141
    activated microglia, 138–140
    astrogliosis, 140–141, 142–143*f*
    cytokines, 141–148
Glial influence, 129–133
    aquaporins (AQPs), 129–130
    astrocytic transforming growth factor-beta
        signaling, 130–133
    cation-chloride cotransporters, 130
    serum albumin, 130–133, 131*f*
Gliosis, 115–116
Glutamate transporters, 170–171

H

High-mobility group box protein 1 (HMGB1),
    163–165
Hippocrates, 1–3, 2*f*

I

Imaging biomarkers, 153–154, 154*f*
Inflammation
    chronic neuroinflammation, 137
    glial cells, 138–141
        activated microglia, 138–140
        astrogliosis, 140–141, 142–143*f*
        cytokines, 141–148
    interleukin-6, 146, 147*f*
    interleukin-10, 143
    interleukin-1 beta, 141–143, 144–145*f*
    migration inhibitory factor, 148
    seizure susceptibility, 137
    targets, 169–170
    transforming growth factor-beta (TGF-β),
        146, 147*f*
    tumor necrosis factor-alpha (TNF-α),
        145–146
Interfascicular cells, 46–47
Interleukin-6, 146, 147*f*
Interleukin-10, 143
Interleukin-1 beta, 141–143, 144–145*f*

J

Jackson, John Hughlings, 12–14, 14*f*

K

Korean War data, 31–32
Krause, Fedor, 19, 20*f*

L

Language functions, localization of, 7–9, 8*f*
Lateral fluid percussion injury (LFPI), 115
Levetiracetam studies, 70
Localization-related epilepsy, 17–24, 18*f*
Location of lesions, 38

M

Magnesium study, 70
Magnetic resonance imaging (MRI), 81–82
Marmarou model, 93, 94*f*
McEwen, William, 14–17, 16*f*
Medial temporal lobe epilepsy (MTLE), 83
Medico-chirurgical neurologist, 61
Meningocerebral cicatrix, 56, 59–60
Mesial temporal sclerosis (MTS), 83
Middle ages, 3–4, 4*f*
Migration inhibitory factor, 148
Military injuries, 29–34
Minozac, 163, 164–165*f*
Montreal Neurological Institute (MNI), 61
Mossy fiber sprouting, 115, 116*f*
Motor functions localization, 9–12, 11*f*

N

Neurological disease, glial alterations in, 52–53
Neurology, 12–17
Neurosurgery, 12–17
Nineteenth century war data, 29

O

Oligodendroglia, 49–52, 51–52*f*, 53*t*

P

Penetrating ballistic-like brain injury (PBBI),
    94–95, 108–109
    ballistic shock wave, 94, 95*f*
    projectiles, 94–95, 95*f*
Penfield, Wilder, 43–52, 44*f*, 45*t*, 56–63,
    58–60*f*, 62*f*
Perineuronal satellites, 50–51
Perivascular satellites, 50–51
Phenytoin studies, 68, 69*f*
Postinjury weight loss, 155
Posttraumatic epilepsy (PTE)
    blast-induced traumatic brain injury (bTBI),
        110
    clinical trials of
        carbamazepine study, 68
        Levetiracetam studies, 70

magnesium study, 70
  perspective, 71
  phenytoin studies, 68, 69f
  valproate study, 69–70
  Vietnam prophylaxis program, 67
controlled cortical impact (CCI) injury
    model, 108, 109f
cortical localization, 7–12
  language functions, localization of, 7–9,
    8f
  motor functions localization, 9–12, 11f
epidemiology of
  civilian injuries, 34–36, 35t, 36f
  clinical heterogeneity, 38–39
  Korean War data, 31–32
  location of lesions, 38
  military injuries, 29–34
  natural history, 38–39
  Nineteenth century war data, 29
  other more recent war data, 33–34
  overview, 29–39
  risk factors, 36–37, 36t
  sports-related concussions, 37
  Vietnam War data, 32–33
  World War I data, 29–31
  World War II data, 31
fluid percussion injury (FPI), 105, 106–107t,
    107f
Foerster, Otfrid, 20–24, 22–23f
hippocrates, 1–3, 2f
Jackson, John Hughlings, 12–14, 14f
Krause, Fedor, 19, 20f
localization-related epilepsy, 17–24, 18f
McEwen, William, 14–17, 16f
middle ages, 3–4, 4f
neurology, 12–17
neuropathology of
  cicatrix, 53–56
  Glasgow Coma Scale, 63t
  histopathology, 63–64
  neurological disease, glial alterations in,
    52–53
  oligodendroglia, 49–52, 51–52f,
    53t
  Penfield, Wilder, 43–52, 44f, 45t, 56–63,
    58–60f, 62f
  Sherrington, Charles S., 44–45, 46f
  traumatic brain injury (TBI), 63–64
  Whipple, Allen O., 45–46, 47f
neurosurgery, 12–17
overview, 1–24
penetrating ballistic-like brain injury
    (PBBI), 108–109

renaissance, 3–4, 4f
surgical approaches to epilepsy, 4–7
surgical treatment of
  case example, 84–89, 86–88f
  modern series of, 81–84, 84–85f
  perspective, 89
  Walker, Arthur Earl, 73–78, 75f, 77f,
    79–80f
  20th century, 17–24
  trephination to craniotomy, 4–7
  undercut traumatic brain injury, 106–107t,
    110–111
  weight drop injury (WDI) model, 108
Preclinical posttraumatic epilepsy research,
    173–176
Primary blast-induced traumatic brain injury
    (bTBI), 96
  Shock tubes, 96, 96f
Protein biomarkers, 154–155

R
Radical operation, 59–60
Rapamycin, 158–159, 159f
Reactive astrocytes, 115–116
Renaissance, 3–4, 4f

S
Satellites, 46–47
Seizure susceptibility, 137
Serum albumin, 130–133, 131f
Sherrington, Charles S., 44–45, 46f
Shock tubes, 96, 96f
Shohami model, 93
Sodium selenate, 159–160
Spontaneous electrocorticograms, 79f
Sports-related concussions, 37

T
Temporal lobe epilepsy (TLE), 84
Therapeutic targets
  astrocyte targets, 170–173
    aquaporin-4, 171–172
    glutamate transporters, 170–171
    other astrocyte targets, 172–173
  inflammation targets, 169–170
  potential therapeutic targets, 169–173
  preclinical posttraumatic epilepsy research,
    173–176
Tight junctions, 127–129, 128–129f
Transforming growth factor-beta (TGF-β),
    146, 147f

Traumatic brain injury (TBI), 1, 63–64,
119–126, 121*f*
controlled cortical impact (CCI) injury,
91–92, 92*f*
fluid percussion injury (FPI), 91, 92*f*
penetrating ballistic-like brain injury
(PBBI), 94–95
ballistic shock wave, 94, 95*f*
projectiles, 94–95, 95*f*
primary blast-induced traumatic brain injury
(bTBI), 96
Shock tubes, 96, 96*f*
undercut traumatic brain injury, 97, 97*f*
weight drop injury (WDI), 92–93
Feeney model, 93, 93*f*
Marmarou model, 93, 94*f*
Shohami model, 93
Treatment trials, 157*t*
baicalein, 156
brivaracetam, 158
ceftriaxone, 158
rapamycin, 158–159, 159*f*
sodium selenate, 159–160
Tumor necrosis factor-alpha (TNF-α),
145–146
Two-hit injury models, 160–165
atipamezole (ATI), 161–163, 162–163*f*

cannabinoid type-1 (CB1) receptor
signaling, 160, 161*f*
high-mobility group box protein 1
(HMGB1), 163–165
minozac, 163, 164–165*f*

U
Undercut traumatic brain injury, 97, 97*f*,
106–107*t*, 110–111

V
Valproate study, 69–70
Vietnam prophylaxis program, 67
Vietnam War data, 32–33

W
Walker-Warburg syndrome, 73–74
Weight drop injury (WDI), 92–93
Feeney model, 93, 93*f*
Marmarou model, 93, 94*f*
model, 108
Shohami model, 93
Whipple, Allen O., 45–46, 47*f*
World War I data, 29–31
World War II data, 31